ANIMAL INGREDIENTS **A TO Z**

PREFACE BY CAROL J. ADAMS • INTRODUCTION BY BRUCE FRIEDRICH

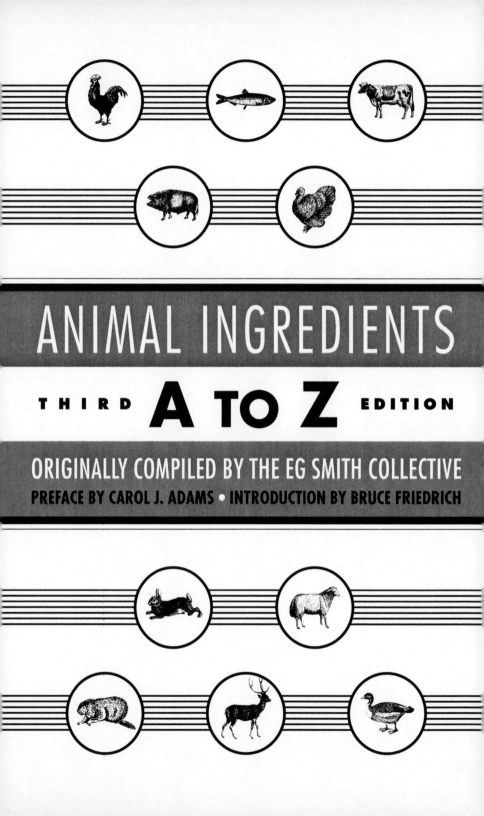

ANIMAL INGREDIENTS

THIRD **A TO Z** EDITION

ORIGINALLY COMPILED BY THE EG SMITH COLLECTIVE
PREFACE BY CAROL J. ADAMS • INTRODUCTION BY BRUCE FRIEDRICH

ANIMAL INGREDIENTS **A TO Z**

© 1997 E.G. Smith Press
First Edition 1995
Second edition 1997
Third edition 2004

ISBN: 1-902593-81-2

AK Press
674-A 23rd Street
Oakland, CA 94612 USA
www.akpress.org

AK Press
PO Box 12766
Edinburgh, Eh8 9YE
Scotland
www.akuk.com

Cover and page design: JONR JONRESH@VIPERPRESS.COM

A catalog record for this title is available from the Library of Congress.

Printed in Canada on 100% Recycled Paper.

The E.G. Smith collective has made every effort to check and double-check all the information contained within for accuracy. To the best of our knowledge, all the information is accurate. The writers, publishers, and/or retailers of this book make no guarantees or claims to the information within.

Sometimes it is good to remind ourselves why we care whether something has whey or lanolin or royal jelly or pepsin in it.

We have learned, through videos like *Meet your Meat*, books like Eric Schlosser's *Fast Food Nation*, and organizations like Farm Sanctuary, that nonhumans are living and dying in unspeakable ways. ... Unspeakable ways that must be spoken about and challenged so that they can be ended.

By the time cosmetics, foods, or clothing are made containing an animal ingredient, the specific nonhuman whose secretion or body has become that ingredient has thoroughly disappeared from view and from consciousness. In *The Sexual Politics of Meat*, I call this process of the disappearance of the nonhuman the structure of the absent referent.

Because of the structure of the absent referent it is difficult to connect nonhumans to the ingredients that they, or their secretions, have become. Nonhumans must be made absent conceptually to enable the consumption and use of their fragmented body parts or secretions.

Because of the absent referent, we encounter "whey" not cows, "lanolin" not sheep, "royal jelly" not bees, and "pepsin" not hogs.

Generally only 50 percent of a slaughtered nonhuman's body is used as "meat." What happens to the remaining 50 percent? It has been dispersed into other products.

Rendering is the process that makes that other half disappear. Rendering is the life support system of the slaughterhouse.

Every rendered part of a nonhuman that is bought as a product rewards, upholds, ratifies the slaughterhouse.

To have a conceptual understanding that nonhumans disappear to enable their consumption as food or as a product is one thing. To act on that understanding is another.

When we decide to say "no" to slaughtering, "no" to flesh eating and dairy consumption, we want also to say "no" to rendering, to the scattering of nonhumans' bodies hither and thither. We want to restore the absent referent. Restoring the absent referent involves the balancing of new truths against old lies, of new information against old products.

Animal Ingredients A to Z is an indispensable resource for new truths and new information. The E.G. Smith Collective has looked through the grocery store, the cosmetic store, the clothing store, they have looked into cars and at the coating on fruit, they have asked companies about teas and "natural flavorings" and found the scattered body parts of nonhumans. The E. G. Smith Collective has restored the absent referent. They help us make what is absent, present — present at least in our minds — so that we can enact a political statement, the boycott.

We can boycott the slaughterhouse and its partner, the rendering industry.

We can boycott the products that arise from the use of nonhumans.

And how do we explain to others who see us looking at the fine print of ingredients?

We say we are trying to do the least harm possible.

We say that changing the world begins with changing the things we make use of in everyday life.

We say that because nonhumans are present to us we don't want to use their body parts or products.

In rejecting products arising from inhumane practices, we are in good company. Consumers have rejected sugar and cotton that was produced by slave states before the Civil War; products from South Africa when apartheid granted the minority whites complete political and economic control; California grapes because they had been harvested by non-unionized farm workers, and clothing imported from sweat shops.

What we are doing is healthy political action on behalf of beings who have been deemed outside the concern of the political sphere.

Why do we care whether something has whey or lanolin or royal jelly or pepsin in it?

Because we want to live lives of integrity.

Because we understand the power of the boycott — of acting individually for a political purpose.

Because we wish to restore the absent referent.

Because in a world that socializes us to be unthinking consumers, we are educating ourselves to refuse to consume.

If we think that our individual actions don't matter, then we absent ourselves from being part of a collective challenge to the use of nonhumans, we absent ourselves from the act of boycotting.

The success of earlier editions of *Animal Ingredients A to Z* reminds us all of something — we are not alone.

Thank you for caring, acting, and changing how we consume.

Carol J. Adams is the author of The Sexual Politics of Meat: A Feminist-Vegetarian Critical Theory, The Pornography of Meat, Living Among Meat Eaters: The Vegetarian' Survival Guide *and several other books. Visit her website at* www.caroljadams.com.

Congratulations!

If you're looking at a list of animal ingredients, it's a safe bet that you're trying to root them all out of your diet. Good for you!

When I became a vegan 15 years ago, it was for environmental and social justice reasons: I had just read Frances Moore Lappé's *Diet for a Small Planet* and didn't want to continue to consume gluttonously, pollute the environment, and steal grain and soybeans and other crops from people who were starving in the developing world. At that point, I wasn't too worried about some modicum of whey or casein or whatever other ingredients fell in the "less than 2 percent" section of the bread or cereal label. I avoided more than 99 percent of animal ingredients, and I was comfortable with that.

Then about 10 years ago, I read *Christianity and the Rights of Animals* by Rev. Andrew Linzey and came to the realization that we should no more consume other animals than we should be consuming other human beings. When we eat animal products, we are consuming corpses. What's more, we're consuming the corpses of animals whose range of emotion is every bit as varied as ours and who feel pain in exactly the same way we do. Apologies to Shakespeare (and Shylock), but if you prick them, the other animals bleed, just as we do; they're made of flesh, blood, and bones, just as we are. That we call other animal flesh "meat" and our flesh, which is exactly the same, "muscle" and "fat" does not change reality: Eating meat means eating corpses. And as far as I'm concerned, corpses should be buried or cremated, not cooked up and consumed.

Of course, there are many other arguments for the elimination of animal products from our diets, but if you're reading this booklet, you're probably as aware of them as I am, and if you're perusing a list of animal ingredients, it's a safe bet that you're trying to root them all out of your diet, cosmetics, and so on. Good for you!

Adopting a vegan diet means saying no to cruelty to animals and environmental destruction and yes to compassion and good health. Going vegan is, I'm convinced, the best thing that you can do for the animals, yourself, and the Earth.

So if adopting a vegan diet is the best thing that you can do, then influencing others must come in a close second. And that's where things become a bit dicey for those of us who are morally and aesthetically revolted by the idea of consuming even small bits of animal corpses! Because although we want to get every last speck of animal parts out of every last thing that we wear or put into our body, it's not possible to be completely pure, and attempting it can, in some very real and frequent circumstances, actually hurt animals—which is, of course, the exact opposite of what we're trying to accomplish as vegans.

So this is PETA's plea for patience and tolerance: Please, don't alienate would-be vegans by examining the food in their cupboards or refrigerators. Don't make veganism seem oh-so-difficult, as though we spend all our time reading labels and demanding that restaurant servers go back and read the label on the bag of veggie burgers. After all, veganism is about joy and life, and it should not be painted as drudgery.

PETA wants to show people that veganism is easy and mainstream because that's what is best for animals. Sadly, some people already perceive vegans as "extreme," "radical," and "difficult." Instead of squabbling about some almost nonexistent ingredient, in public situations we should be positive and not pretend that even "pure" vegan food doesn't come with its quota of rat hairs allowed by law, isn't processed using electricity that destroys habitat, isn't delivered in gas-fueled vehicles, and so on.

Everything that we eat involves some degree of animal suffering; our goal is to vigorously reduce that suffering. Frankly, some not-quite-vegan food is more vegan than the streets and tires we drive on, the houses we live in, the petroleum products we use, and many other animal-based products that we unwittingly consume on a daily basis.

Remember, if you give a server in a restaurant the third degree or spend all your time with your parents telling them that this, that, or the other is not vegan on the basis of some infinitesimal ingredient that they've never even heard of, you'll inadvertently be transforming your noble desire to promote compassion into the message that being compassionate is an arduous chore. Someone who might have been swayed to your way of thinking will come away with the impression that veganism is too difficult.

In that event, your desire to withdraw support for, say, 1/10,000th of the suffering of an animal will have a direct result in the suffering of the thousands of animals that that person will now consume as a result of your actions. The animals need you to take this issue seriously and make advocacy every bit as important as, or even more important than, personal purity.

We are not saying that you shouldn't try to wipe all the nonvegan ingredients out of your life. What we are saying is that if you're that worried about these issues, please find out which items are 100 percent vegan but don't make a fuss over them; and when you eat out, call ahead to make sure that the restaurant that you're patronizing has vegan options. With a bit of advance planning, you can adhere to a lifestyle that is as vegan as you like, and others will be able to have a pleasant time in your company without feeling that your life is filled with nothing but worry over ingredients.

Thanks so much for taking the vegan journey. Bon voyage!

Bruce Friedrich is director of vegan outreach for People for the Ethical Treatment of Animals (PETA).

For us, the past two years have consisted of a painstaking collection of data and research. As before, space constraints have required us to exclude a lot of helpful articles in their entirety. However, we have taken the cold hard facts of these articles and included them here. A complete listing of these articles can be found in the back of this book and we do recommend that you take the time to dig them up and read them.

We have attempted not to write an animal rights book, but a clear, concise reference manual. Our views on animal rights should be self-evident.

As thorough and complete as we have attempted to be, no one list on the subject can ever be considered absolutely complete. Industry is creating new ingredients every day. With this in mind, you will find a bit more explanation in this edition to aid in making the many educated guesses that a vegan is faced with on a day-to-day basis. Starting with some nutrition facts to help dispel myths about how unhealthy not eating meat is, we go on to bring fact to the fiction (or non-fiction) of many rumors that we have all heard many times and even some that we were surprised to hear. Regardless of how outrageous a reported rumor would sound, we went to lengths in checking it out through the FDA, the manufacturer, and wherever else we could find the information.

Most of the FDA boards that review products and make policies regarding their labeling are typically all ex-food product executives. This fact alone makes the FDA an unreliable source of information. In the current political climate, and with capitalism at it's strongest, the FDA is often pressured to make decisions biased to the manufacturers' liking. Often a good deal, if not all, of the research on any given product is done by the manufacturers themselves. So the bias should be obvious. Food manufacturers also use tactics (coined by Procter & Gamble) like contributing large amounts of capital to key members of the Congress to gain lobbying power.

The manufacturers were not helpful in finding out specifics on particular products as they went to every extreme to protect their products and maintain the salability to all consumers. Of course, any food product from any major manufacturer (i.e. Proctor & Gamble, General Mills, etc.) will have most likely

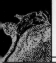

been tested on animals regardless of whether or not there are animal-derived products in it.

It is best to buy food products from the smaller companies out there, or try your hand at organic gardening. Unfortunately these two alternatives are not always feasible depending on where you live. That's why we've worked so hard to pull a book like this together.

In researching this book we have been astounded at some of the inventive places animal products can pop up. Our diets have changed in the course of compiling the information here, as we were surprised to find many ingredients that we were eating contained animal products.

We have continued to be as thorough and correct as possible. All information contained in this publication is from reliable sources, all of which are documented at the end. Most have been double checked with our own resources.

The E.G. Smith Press Collective

The purpose of this pamphlet isn't to preach about why you shouldn't eat animals and how animals are tortured because of society's consumption of them. It has been compiled as a working reference for those who are most likely vegan, and who wonder if Dihydroxyethyl Soyamine Dioleate in their favorite potato chips is vegan (which it isn't).

This pamphlet is comprised of several different articles from all over the country. There were a lot of things that we had collected that we wanted to include but due to the space constraints we were forced to carefully select articles that stayed consistent with the original goal we had set out to accomplish.

The Possibly Animal Derived list in this pamphlet requires some explanation. This is a myriad of ingredients that fit into two categories. The first is ingredients that are most likely animal derived, but no confirmation has been given by the manufacturer(s). The other is ingredients that in some cases are animal derived, but not always. Usually it is best to use your judgment. Lecithin for example will say Soy-Lecithin if it is not derived from animals; on the other hand some ingredients offer no clue to their origins. It is usually best to avoid most of the products listed in this section, just to be safe.

The booklet focuses mainly on food, but it also extends somewhat into shampoos and other products that even people of the meat-eating culture wouldn't normally eat. We have tried to be as thorough and correct as possible. All the information contained in this publication is from reliable sources, all of which are documented at the end, and most have been double checked with our own resources.

The E.G. Smith Press Collective

People just turning vegan as well as veteran vegans are faced daily with deciding if a rumor is true. We all know the story…I have a friend whose father's drinking buddy works in the such and such factory and says they use beef blood as a processing agent.

Here we try to dispel some common myths, give a brief history on the origin of the word vegetarian, offer some facts about those symbols declaring something Kosher, the truth about the wax on the produce stories, and offer some alternatives to eggs.

In brief, this chapter is a compilation of information we really felt should be included, but didn't really have a category for it. It also turned out to be one of the most interesting chapters to work on.

WHERE DID THE TERM "VEGETARIAN" COME FROM?

The term "Vegetarian" was coined in 1847. It was first formally used on September 30th of that year by Joseph Brotherton and others, at Northwood Villa in Kent, England. The occasion was the inaugural meeting of the Vegetarian Society of the United Kingdom.

The word was derived from the Latin "vegetus," meaning whole, sound, fresh, lively; (it should not be confused with "vegetable-arian—a mythical human whom some imagine subsisting entirely on vegetables but no nuts, fruits, grains etc!)

Prior to 1847, non-meat eaters were generally known as "Pythagoreans" or adherents of the "Pythagorean System," after the ancient Greek "vegetarian" Pythagoras.

The original definition of "vegetarian" was "with or without eggs or dairy products" and that definition is still used by the Vegetarian Society today. However, most vegetarians in India exclude eggs from their diet, as did those in the classical Mediterranean lands, such as Pythagoras.

COMMON MYTHS

CHEWING GUM: Some chewing gums contain glycerin/glycerine (see pg. 38). Wrigley's gum contains a vegetarian source of glycerin(e).

ENVELOPES: Apparently most envelopes have synthetic glue on them, not an animal or fish based glue.

HEINZ CATSUP: Heinz has officially denied that they use beef blood as part of their "Natural Flavoring"(see pg. 33) in their catsup. They claim that there are no animal ingredients at all in their "Natural Flavoring." E.G. Smith is still unconvinced.

MAPLE SYRUP: Yes, rumors abound about maple syrup containing pork fat. The US vegan society has checked all known sources and found that they are all suitable for vegans.

OLESTRA, MAX, OLEAN: (see pg. 43) By time this book is printed Olestra, which is sold under the brand name OLEAN (Procter & Gamble), and MAX (Frito-Lay), will have either hit the international market by storm or completely have been rejected due to the harmful side effects this fake fat has on the human body. Without going into much detail on Olestra itself, it will suffice to say that it is not vegan. Although Proctor & Gamble won't tell us exactly what is in it, it has been confirmed to contain FATTY ACIDS (see pg. 36) and is therefore not vegan. E.G. Smith Press can provide additional up to date information on the harmful fat substitute, Olestra, upon request.

POSTAGE STAMPS: These do not contain animal or fish glue.

SUGAR: The popular rumor says that cane sugar is processed through gelatin. This is untrue. Some cane sugars are processed using boneblack as a decolorant (see Chapter 2). The process is similar but not the same. Gelatin is boiled skin, tendons, ligaments or bones, while boneblack is actually charcoaled – at any rate, it is not suitable for vegans. We contacted several popular cane sugar manufacturers and they all confirmed the use of boneblack in their processes. We recommend contacting the manufacturer directly to inquire whether or not their particular brand of sugar is vegan. In the UK, Tate and Lyle and Billingtons sugars are free of animal substances. British Sugar, trading as Silver Spoon (the largest UK supplier), state that their white sugar is vegan but they cannot guarantee their brown sugars are, as some bone charcoal may be used by their suppliers.

TEA: Rumors have sprung up claiming that Tetley and Lipton use animal products (or blood, in particular) as coloring in their teas. Tetley was very kind in their response, being very specific. However, Lipton was less specific and a little bit harder to get a straight answer from. They do confirm that there are no animal products used in their coloring. However, they refrain from being specific as to the Natural Flavors (see pg. 42) part of their ingredients list. E.G. Smith's position on this is wary, we suggest you judge for yourself based on their response(s).

OUR ORIGINAL LETTER TO LIPTON
Dear Lipton,
There are rumors abound that you use animal products in the coloring of your teas. Many vegetarians and health conscious alike, would be interested in the truth in this rumor. Do you, in fact, use any animal or animal-derived products in any of your teas? Please be specific.
Thank You,
E.G. Smith Project

THEIR VAGUE RESPONSE

Dear E.G. Smith:

The flavor of the tea in all our products is derived from the tealeaves during the brewing process. All of our other ingredients are FDA approved before we market a product. I hope this information is helpful and thanks for your interest in Lipton!

Your friends at Lipton

OUR REPLY

Thank you for your prompt response. However, "FDA approved" does include animal-derived products. We aren't asking disclosure of the actual ingredients, simply, are there any animal-derived ingredients in any of your teas, and if so which ones?

Thanks again,

The E.G. Smith Project

LIPTON'S FINAL ANSWER

Dear E.G. Smith Project, I have checked with our staff and we do not use animal products in the coloring of our tea (leaf or powdered). I hope this is helpful.

Your friends at Lipton

ON KOSHER...

Kosher means that a particular food is made according to a complex set of Jewish dietary laws. Does not imply VEGAN in any case. Does not imply Vegetarian in any case. Even KOSHER products containing milk products may contain some types of animals that are not considered "meat."

A common misconception is checking if a food is Kosher to determine whether or not it is vegan. The following are some of the Kosher designations with their meanings.

D: Dairy

DE: Dairy Equipment (no actual dairy in ingredients, equipment may have been used previously in the manufacture of products containing dairy)

P: Passover Kosher for all year including Passover (Note: "P" NEVER designates pareve)

PAREVE: Non-dairy

KEEP THIS IN MIND:

PAREVE/PARVE: One category in KOSHER dietary laws. Made without meat or milk products or their derivatives. Eggs and true fish are pareve, shellfish are not.

NONDAIRY: Does not have enough percentage of milk fat to be called dairy. May actually contain milk or milk derivatives.

NONMEAT: Made without meat. May include eggs, milk, or cheese. Sometimes even includes animal fats, seafood, fish, or fowl.

WAXED PRODUCE

What looks good sells. Several supermarkets across the country are using wax and such on their fruits and vegetables to make them look more appealing. Some of these visual enhancers are animal based.

"The Food and Drug Administration has registered several categories of waxes for topical use on apples, avocados, oranges, lemons, limes, grapefruit, melons, peaches, pineapples, passion fruits, cucumbers, eggplants, peppers, pumpkins, rutabagas, squash, tomatoes, sweet potatoes, turnips, and other fruits and vegetables. The produce-packing industry argues that waxes, which often contain chemical fungicides, are needed to reduce shrinkage from moisture loss and to inhibit the growth of molds and fungus. According to FDA regulations, retailers must label waxed produce; however, nobody does this, and the law is unenforced. The types of waxes currently in use on produce are:

SUITABLE FOR VEGANS

CARNAUBA WAX. Obtained from the wax palm of Brazil, carnauba is the hardest of the natural waxes. It is used widely in floor waxes, polishes, and lubricants.

PARAFFIN. A derivative of petroleum, paraffin is flammable and insoluble in water. It is used to make candles and for many industrial purposes.

CANDELILLA. Obtained from a reed, candelilla is a natural wax that is common in furniture polishes.

POLYETHYLENE. A plastic synthesized from petroleum, polyethylene is manufactured in sheets and films. Its many commercial uses include unbreakable bottles, shower curtains, electrical insulation, pipes, and packaging materials.

NOT SUITABLE FOR VEGANS

SHELLAC. Obtained from the bodies of the female scale insect Tachardia lacca, shellac is used as varnish, as a coating on wood and plaster, in electrical insulation, and in sealing wax,

OLEIC ACID. Obtained from vegetable oils, animal fats, or synthesized from petroleum, oleic acid is used in industrial lubricants.

TALLOW. Obtained from the tissues and fatty deposits of animals, especially cattle and sheep, tallow is used in floor waxes, soap, candles, and as a lubricant.

If the produce is not labeled it is impossible to tell what is used on the produce you're eating, if any at all. These waxes cannot be washed off produce. If you want to avoid eating waxes, peel any produce that is waxed.

The Complete Book of Juicing by Michael Murray, ND (Prima Publishing, 1992), says essentially the same thing. However, Dr. Murray does offer some advice on reducing exposure to waxes:

1. Buy organic produce.

2. Try to buy local produce that is in season. Produce imported into the US is more likely to contain excessive levels of pesticides as well as pesticides that have been banned in the US.

3. Soak produce in a mild solution of additive-free soap like pure castille soap to remove surface pesticide residues, fungicides, and fertilizers.

4. Peel off the skin or remove the outer layer of leaves.

To find out more information on the rules and regulations the FDA has set for this practice you can call the Food & Drug Administration and request a copy of docket number 90N-0361 "Food Labeling: Declaration of Ingredients."

WHAT CAN BE SUBSTITUTED FOR EGGS?

• A company called Ener-G makes a powdered egg-substitute that they claim is a suitable replacement for eggs in cooking. It costs about $5.00 (US) for the equivalent of 9 or 10 dozen eggs, and it contains no animal products.

• 2 oz of soft tofu can be blended with some water and added to substitute for an egg to add consistency.

• One Tbsp flax seeds (found in natural food stores) with 3 Tbsp water can be blended for 2 to 3 minutes, or boiled for 10 minutes or until desired consistency is achieved to substitute for one egg.

• 1/ 2 mashed banana for one egg.

• 1/4 cup applesauce or pureed fruit for one egg.

• 1 Tsp soy flour plus 1 Tbsp water to substitute for one egg.

Has anyone ever told you that "you're going to die of malnutrition"? How about "you have to eat meat for a balanced diet"? The fact of the matter is that meat is not healthy and vegetarians and vegans are usually healthier people, who suffer from fewer cases of heart disease, fewer cases of cancer, and fewer long-term health problems. This has been proven time and time again through thousands upon thousands of studies.

This chapter will attempt to give a brief introduction to basic nutrition then move on to explore all of the essential nutrients that a human needs to live a long, healthy life.

We will look at what these nutrients are needed for and how to obtain them from vegetarian sources.

A BRIEF INTRODUCTION TO BASIC NUTRITION

Many people worry that when they stop eating meat and fish, they might be in danger of some nutritional deficiency. This is rarely the case, as all the nutrients you need can easily be obtained from a vegetarian diet. In fact, research shows that in many ways, a vegetarian diet is healthier than that of a typical meat-eater.

Nutrients are usually divided into five classes: carbohydrates, proteins, fats (including oil), vitamins and minerals. We also need fiber and water. All are equally important to our well-being, although they are needed in varying quantities, from about 250g of carbohydrates a day to less than two micrograms of vitamin B12. Carbohydrates, fats and protein are usually called macro-nutrients and the vitamins and minerals are usually called micro-nutrients.

Most foods contain a mixture of nutrients (there are a few exceptions, like pure salt or sugar) but it is convenient to classify them by the main nutrient they provide. Still, it is worth remembering that everything you eat gives you a whole range of essential nutrients.

Meat supplies protein, fat, some B vitamins and minerals (mostly iron, zinc, potassium and phosphorous). Fish, in addition to the above, supplies vitamins A, D, and E, and the mineral iodine. All these nutrients can be easily obtained by vegetarians from other sources.

Women need about 46-50g of protein a day (more if pregnant, lactating or very active), men need about 56-63g (more if very active). Evidence suggests that excessive protein contributes to degenerative diseases.

You may have heard that it is necessary to balance the complementary amino acids in a vegetarian diet. This is not as alarming as it sounds. Amino acids are the units from which proteins are made. There are 21 different ones in all. We can make many of them in our bodies by converting other amino acids, but nine cannot be made. They have to be provided in the diet and so they are called essential amino acids.

Single plant foods do not contain all the essential amino acids we need in the right proportions, but when we mix plant foods together, any deficiency in one is cancelled out by any excess in the other. We mix protein foods all the time, whether we are meat-eaters or vegetarians. It is a normal part of the human way of eating. A few examples are beans on toast, muesli, or rice and peas.

It is now known that the body has a pool of amino acids so that if one meal is deficient, it can be made up from the body's own stores. Because of this, we don't have to worry about complementing amino acids all the time, as long as our diet is generally varied and well-balanced. Even those foods not considered high in protein are adding some amino acids to this pool.

CARBOHYDRATES

Carbohydrates are our main and most important source of energy, and most of them are provided by plant foods. There are three main types: simple sugars, complex carbohydrates or starches and dietary fiber.

The sugars or simple carbohydrates can be found in fruit and ordinary table sugar. Refined sources of sugar are best avoided as they provide energy without any associated fiber, vitamins or minerals and they are also the main cause of dental decay.

Complex carbohydrates are found in cereals/grains (bread, rice, pasta, oats, barley, millet, buckwheat, rye) and some root vegetables, such as potatoes and parsnips. A healthy diet should contain plenty of these starchy foods, as a high intake of complex carbohydrates is now known to benefit health. The unrefined carbohydrates, like wholemeal bread and brown rice are best of all because they contain essential dietary fiber and 13 vitamins.

The World Health Organization recommends that 50-70% of energy should come from complex carbohydrates. The exact amount of carbohydrates that you need depends upon your appetite and also your level of activity. Contrary to previous belief, a slimming diet should not be low in carbohydrates. In fact, starchy foods are very filling in relation to the number of calories that they contain.

Dietary Fiber or non-starch polysaccharide (NSP), as it is now termed, refers to the indigestible part of a carbohydrate food. Fiber can be found in unrefined or wholegrain cereals, fruit (fresh and dried) and vegetables. A good intake of dietary fiber can prevent many digestive problems and protect against diseases like colon cancer and diverticular disease.

FATS & OILS

Too much fat is bad for us, but a little is necessary to keep our tissues in good repair, for the manufacture of hormones and to act as a carrier for some vitamins. Like proteins, fats are made of smaller units, called fatty acids. Two of these fatty acids, linoleic and linolenic acids, are termed essential as they must be provided in the diet. This is no problem as they are widely found in plant foods.

Fats can be either saturated or unsaturated (mono-unsaturated or poly-unsaturated). A high intake of saturated fat can lead to a raised blood cholesterol level and this has been linked to heart disease. Vegetable fats tend to be more unsaturated and this is one of the benefits of a vegetarian diet. Mono-unsaturated fats, such as olive oil or peanut oil, are best used for frying as the poly-unsaturated fats, like sunflower or safflower oil are unstable at high temperatures. Animal fats (including butter and cheese) tend to be more saturated than vegetable fats, with the exception of palm oil, coconut oil and cocoa butter.

VITAMINS

Vitamin is the name for several unrelated nutrients that the body cannot synthesize either at all, or in sufficient quantities. The one thing they have in common is that only small quantities are needed in the diet. The main vegetarian sources are listed below:

Vitamin A (or beta carotene): Red, orange or yellow vegetables like carrots and tomatoes, leafy green vegetables and fruits like apricots and peaches. It is added to most margarines.

B Vitamins: This group of vitamins includes B1 (thiamin), B2 (riboflavin), B3 (niacin), B6 (pyridoxine), B12 (cyanocobalmin), folate, folic acid, pantothenic acid and biotin. All the B vitamins except B12 occur in yeasts and whole cereals (especially wheat germ), nuts & seeds, pulses and green vegetables. Vitamin B12 is the only one that may cause some difficulty, as it is not present in plant foods. Only very tiny amounts of B12 are needed. Vitamin B12 is added to yeast extracts, Soy milks, veggie burgers and some breakfast cereals.

Vitamin C: Fresh fruit, salad vegetables, all leafy green vegetables and potatoes.

Vitamin D: This vitamin is not found in plant foods but humans can make their own when skin is exposed to sunlight, It is also added to most margarines. Vegans who are very young, very old and anyone confined indoors would be wise to take a vitamin D supplement.

Vitamin E: Vegetable oil, whole grain cereals, leafy greens.

Vitamin K: Fresh vegetables, soybean oil, cereals and bacterial synthesis in the intestine.

MINERALS
Minerals perform a variety of jobs in the body. Details of some of the most important minerals (Calcium, Iron, and Zinc) are in the next section.

ALPHABETICAL LISTING OF NUTRIENTS

CALCIUM is for the development and growth of bones and teeth, normal clotting of blood and functioning of muscles. The body can't absorb calcium without Vitamin D. Calcium can be found in: watercress, rhubarb, beets, parsley, spinach, broccoli, Chinese cabbage, raw onions, raw celery, akra/okra, chives, raw cabbage, cucumbers, turnips, zucchini, green beans, squash, artichokes, leafy green vegetables, tap water in hard water areas.

CARBOHYDRATES are for energy, heat and to assist in the absorption of fat-soluble vitamins & calcium. Carbohydrates can be found in: cereals, bread & flour products, dried fruits, dried peas & beans, bananas, sugar, potatoes.

COPPER is for the manufacture of red blood cells, bones, collagen, healing wounds, even creation of RNA (Ribonucleic Acid). Copper can be found in: nuts & beans, dried peas, wheat bran, whole wheat, molasses, mushrooms, avocados, broccoli.

ESSENTIAL FATTY ACIDS limit the formation of excess cholesterol in the blood. They are sources of the prostaglandins, which regulate processes in the smooth muscles. Essential fatty acids can be found in: corn, walnuts, vegetable oils, peanuts, sesame, sunflower & safflower seeds.

FATS are necessary for healthy skin, energy, heat and to assist in the absorption of fat-soluble vitamins and calcium. Fats can be found in: vegetable oils, nuts & nut creams, cooking fats, nut butters, margarine, vegan white fats.

FIBER keeps vascular system in good tone, i.e. prevents troubles in the intestines, veins and arteries. Fiber can be found in: citrus fruits, apples, potatoes, peas, beans, broccoli, carrots and unrefined foods (especially cereals).

FOLIC ACID is used to synthesize and break down amino acids. It also prevents certain kinds of anemia, assists growth and can be found in nuts, grains, oranges, avocados, all green vegetables, yeast extracts.

IODINE is for healthy growth and development. Present in vegetables, but the quantity depends on how rich the soil is in iodine. Sea vegetables are a good source of iodine for vegans. Other sources are: dried beans, asparagus, green veggies, pineapple.

IRON is for proper formation of red blood cells and regulation of body processes. Vegetable sources of iron are not as easily absorbed as animal sources, but a good intake of vitamin C will enhance absorption. Iron can be found in: prunes, whole grain cereals, black treacle, raisins, nuts, leafy green vegetables, sesame seeds, Soy flour, pulses, cocoa, curry powder, wholemeal bread, molasses, dried fruits (especially apricots and figs). Cook in cast iron.

MANGANESE is necessary for strong bones, healthy skin, the proper functioning of muscle and nervous tissue. Manganese can be found in: legumes, nuts, fruits, tea, alfalfa, chlorophyll, wheat germ, whole grains.

NICOTINAMIDE is for healthy digestion, good skin condition, and growth. Nicotinamide can be found in: Soy, peanuts, flour & bread, yeast, rice, pulses, beer.

PROTEIN helps growth and the repair of body tissues. Also for energy, their physical properties may be changed by cooking and food preparation generally. Protein comes from several sources. Nuts: hazels, brazils, almonds, cashews, walnuts, pine kernels etc. Seeds: sesame, pumpkin, sunflower, linseeds. Pulses: peas, beans, lentils, peanuts. Grains/Cereals: wheat (in bread, soy flour, pasta etc), barley, rye, oats, millet, maize (sweetcorn), rice, gluten flour, bakers yeast, brewers yeast. Soy products: tofu, tempeh, textured vegetable protein, veggie burgers, Soy milk.

TRACE ELEMENTS are essential accessories to vital processes and to action of other nutrients. Trace elements can be found in: carrots, watercress, dried apricots, prunes, tomatoes, cabbage, green peas, all green vegetables and margarine.

VITAMIN A is for growth in children, plays a part in the way the eyes receive light, and protects moist surface tissues (bronchial tubes, etc.). Vitamin A can be found in: peppers, parsley, carrots, sweet potatoes, apricots, spinach, mangoes, chives, squash.

VITAMIN B1 (Thiamin) is for growth, appetite, digestion, and the nervous system. Vitamin B1 can be found in: bread and wheat products, pulses, yeast (brewers is best), Brazils and peanuts (uncooked), wheat germ.

VITAMIN B2 (Riboflavin) is for vitality, healthy skin, the release of food energy, growth and good sight. Vitamin B2 can be found in: yeast, lentils, rye, mushrooms, parsley, broccoli tops, green vegetables.

VITAMIN B12 is needed for cell division and blood formation. Plant foods do not contain vitamin B12 except when they are contaminated by microorganisms. Thus, vegans need to look to other sources to get vitamin B12 in their diet. Although the minimum requirement for vitamin B12 is quite small, 1/1,000,000 of a gram (1 microgram) a day for adults, a vitamin B12 deficiency is a very serious problem leading ultimately to irreversible nerve damage. Prudent vegans will include sources of vitamin B12 in their diets. However, vitamin B12 deficiency is actually quite rare even among long-term vegans. Vitamin B12 also aids growth of nerve cells and the prevention of certain kinds of anemia. A deficiency results in pernicious anemia.

The requirement for vitamin B12 is very low. Non-animal sources include Grape-Nuts cereal (1/2 cup supplies the adult RDA) and Red Star T-6635+ nutritional yeast (1-2 teaspoons supplies the adult RDA). It is especially important for pregnant and lactating women, infants, and children to have reliable sources of vitamin B12 in their diets. Other sources include: brewers yeast, bakers yeast, rice bran, wheat germ, sunflower seeds, cornflakes, pinon nuts, soy milk, sesame seeds, brazil nuts, and peanuts. Higher to lower levels found in: edible seaweeds, hijiki and wakame, mushrooms, nutritional yeast, tempeh, miso, syrup, sourdough bread, parsley, beer, cider, wine, yeast, tofu, supplemented fortified foods, some yeast extracts, Soy-based textured vegetable proteins, Soy milks and margarine.

VITAMIN C is famous for healing wounds, prevention of scurvy, boosting the immune system, maintaining stamina, forming strong blood vessels, and aiding resistance to infection. Vitamin C can be found in: bell peppers, guavas, peppers, broccoli, watercress, parsley, radishes, asparagus, brussel sprouts, chives, strawberries, papayas, cantaloupes, oranges, grapefruit.

VITAMIN D builds bones & teeth, prevents the destruction of vitamins C and A, and aids growth. Vitamin D can be found in: mild exposure to sunlight, sunflower seeds, mushrooms,

VITAMIN E is for growth, muscle tissues, and normal reproduction. Possibly retards aging. Vitamin E can be found in: wheat and rice germ, whole wheat grains, soybean oil, leafy greens, nuts and seeds, legumes.

VITAMIN K regulates clotting of blood. Vitamin K can be found in green leafy vegetables.

ZINC plays a major role in many enzyme reactions and in the immune system. It also aids in fighting infections. Zinc can be found in: nuts & seeds, wheat germ, brewers yeast, whole grains, yellow & green veggies, yellow fruits, pumpkin & sesame seeds, lentils, whole grain cereals.

If you don't find the ingredient here, check the Animal Ingredients chapter (chapter 4) or the Possibly Animal Derived chapter (chapter 6) in this book. If you still don't find the ingredient that you're unsure about, try a dictionary or use your best judgment.

ACETATE: Retinol. Vitamin A. Palmitate (see Palmitic Acid). An aliphatic alcohol that can come from fish liver oil (i.e. shark liver oil), egg yolks, butter, lemongrass, wheat germ oil, carotene in carrots, etc., synthetics. In cosmetics, creams, perfumes, hair dyes, vitamins, supplements.

ADRENALINE: From the adrenals of hogs, cattle and sheep. In medicines. Alternatives: synthetics

AFTERBIRTH: Placenta. Placenta Polypeptides Protein. Contains waste matter eliminated by the fetus. Derived from the uterus of slaughtered animals. Animal placenta is widely used in skin creams, shampoos, masks, etc. Doesn't remove wrinkles. Alternatives: kelp, vegetable oils.

ALBUMEN: Egg Albumen. Albumin. In eggs, milk, muscles, blood and in many vegetable tissues and fluids. In cosmetics, albumin is usually derived from egg whites. May cause allergic reactions. In cakes, cookies, candies, other foods. Egg whites sometimes used in "clearing" wines.

ALBUMIN: See *Albumen*.

ALIPHATIC ALCOHOL: See *Acetate*.

ALLANTOIN: A uric acid from cows and most mammals. Also in many plants (especially comfrey). In cosmetics, especially creams & lotions, and used in the treatment of wounds and skin ulcers.

AMBERGRIS: From sperm whale intestines. Used as a fixative in perfumes and as a flavoring in foods and beverages. (US regulations currently prohibit the use of ingredients derived from marine mammals.) Alternatives: synthetic and vegetable fixatives.

AMINO ACIDS: Animal or plant sources. In cosmetics, vitamins, supplements, shampoos, etc.

AMINOSUCCINATE ACID: DL and L forms. Aspartic Acid. Can be animal or plant (i.e. molasses) source. Is a nonessential amino acid. In creams and ointments. Sometimes synthesized for commercial purposes.

AMYLASE: An enzyme prepared from the pancreas of hogs. In cosmetics and medicines.

ANIMAL BONES: Bone Meal. In some fertilizers, some vitamins and supplements as a source of calcium, also in toothpastes. Alternatives: plant mulch, vegetable compost, dolomite, clay, vegetarian vitamins.

ANIMAL OILS AND FATS: In foods, cosmetics, etc. Highly allergenic. Plant derivatives are superior. Alternatives: olive oil, wheat germ oil, coconut oil, almond oil, safflower oil, etc.

ARACHIDONIC ACID: A liquid unsaturated fatty acid occurring in the liver, brain, glands, and fat of animals. Generally isolated from the liver. In skin creams and lotions to soothe eczema and rashes.

ASPARTIC ACID: See *Aminosuccinate Acid.*

ASPIC: An industry alternative for gelatin. Is made from clarified meat, fish or vegetable stocks and gelatin.

BEE POLLEN: Collected from the legs of bees. Causes allergic reactions in some people. In supplements, shampoos, toothpaste, deodorants. Too concentrated for human use.

BEE PRODUCTS: From bees. For bees. Bees are selectively bred. Culls are killed. A cheap sugar is substituted for their stolen honey and millions die as a result. Their legs are often torn off by pollen-collecting trap doors.

BEESWAX: Obtained from the honeycomb of bees. Very cheap and traditional, but harmful to the skin. Some companies won't use beeswax as it doesn't permit the skin to breathe. In lipsticks and many other cosmetics, especially face creams, lotions, mascaras, eye creams and shadows, makeup bases, nail whiteners, etc. Used in making candles, crayons and polishes. Alternatives: Paraffin; vegetable oils and fats; ceresin, made from the mineral ozokerite (replaces beeswax in candle making); carnauba wax from the Brazilian palm tree (used in many cosmetics and in the manufacture of rubber, phonograph records, in waterproofing and writing inks); synthetic beeswax.

BENZOIC ACID: In almost all vertebrates and in berries. In mouthwashes, deodorants, creams, aftershave lotions, perfumes, foods, and beverages. Alternatives: gum benzoin (tincture) from the aromatic balsamic resin from trees grown in China, Sumatra, Thailand and Cambodia.

BETA CAROTENE: Provitamin A. Carotene. Found in many animal tissues and in all plants. Used as a coloring in cosmetics and in the manufacture of Vitamin A.

BIOTIN: Vitamin H. Vitamin B Factor. In every living cell and in larger amounts in milk and yeast. Used in cosmetics, shampoos, creams. Alternatives: plant sources.

BLOOD: This should be obvious but if it isn't.... From any slaughtered animal. Used in cheese making, foam rubber, intravenous feedings, medicines, and as adhesive in plywood. Possibly in foods as lecithin (see choline bitartrate). Alternatives: synthetics, plant sources.

BOAR BRISTLES: Hair from wild or captive hogs. In "natural" toothbrushes, hairbrushes, bath brushes, cosmetic brushes and shaving brushes. Alternatives: vegetable fibers, nylon.

BONE ASH: Bone Earth. The ash of burned bones, used as a fertilizer, in making ceramics and in cleaning and polishing compounds.

BONEBLACK: Bone Charcoal. A black pigment containing about 10% charcoal made by roasting bones in an airtight container. Used in aquarium filters and in refining cane sugar. In eye shadows, polishes.

BONE CHARCOAL: See *Boneblack.*

BONE EARTH: See *Bone Ash.*

BONE MEAL: See *Animal Bones.*

CALCIFEROL: Vitamin D. Ergocalciferol (Vitamin D2, Ergosterol, provitamin D2, Calciferol). Vitamin D3. Vitamin D can come from fish-liver oil, eggs, milk, butter. Vitamin D2 is made by irradiating ergosterol, a provitamin from plants or yeast. Vitamin D3 is from fish-liver oil. In creams, lotions, other cosmetics, vitamins. Alternatives: sunshine, plant sources, synthetics.

CALCIUM CARBONATE: Calcite. Aragonite. A white powder or colorless, crystalline compound found mainly in limestone, marble and chalk, bones, teeth, shells and plant ash.

CALCIUM HYDROXIDE: Slaked lime, a white crystalline compound prepared by the action of water on Calcium Oxide (see), used in making alkalies, bleaching powder, etc.

CALCIUM OXIDE: a white soft, caustic solid, prepared by heating Calcium Carbonate (see); lime: used in making mortar and plaster, and in ceramics.

CALCIUM PHOSPHATE: Any number of phosphates of calcium found in bones, teeth, and other animal tissues and used in medicine and in the manufacture of enamels, glass, cleaning agents, etc.

CAPRYLIC ACID: Can come from cow or goat milk. Also from palm and coconut oil, other plant oils. In perfumes, soaps.

CARBAMIDE: Urea. Imidazolidinyl Urea. Uric Acid. Found in urine and other body fluids. Also produced synthetically. In deodorants, ammoniated dentifrices, mouthwashes, hair colorings, hand creams, lotions, shampoos, etc. Used to "brown" baked goods such as pretzels.

CARMINE: Cochineal. Carminic Acid. E120. Red pigment from the crushed female cochineal insect. Reportedly 70,000 beetles may be killed to produce one pound of this red dye. Used in cosmetics, shampoos, red applesauce and other foods. May cause allergic reactions. Alternatives: beet juice, no known toxicity (used in powders, rouges, shampoos); alkanet root, from the root of an herblike tree, no known toxicity (used as a red dye for inks, wines, lip balms, etc. and can be combined to make a copper or blue coloring).

CARMINIC ACID: See *Carmine.*

CAROTENE: See *Beta Carotene.*

CASEIN: Caseinogen. Milk protein. In "non-dairy" creamers, many cosmetics, hair preparations, beauty masks. Alternatives: soy protein, vegetable milks.

CASEINOGEN: See *Casein.*

CASTOR: Castoreum. From muskrat and beaver genitals. Used in perfumes and incense. Castor oil comes from the castor bean and is used in many cosmetics. Alternatives: synthetics, plant sources.

CASTOREUM: See *Castor.*

CATGUT: Tough cord or thread made from the intestines of sheep, horses, etc. Used for surgical sutures and for stringing tennis rackets and musical instruments, etc. Alternatives: nylon & other man-made fibers.

CETYL ALCOHOL: Cetyl Lactate. Cetyl Myristate. Cetyl Palmitate. Ceteth-1, -2, etc. Wax found in spermaceti (see) from sperm whales or dolphins. Used in lipsticks, mascaras, nail polish removers, hand lotions, cream, rouges and many other cosmetics, shampoos, hair lacquers and other hair products, deodorants, antiperspirants. (US regulations currently prohibit the use of ingredients derived from marine mammals.) Alternatives: vegetable cetyl alcohol (i.e. coconut), synthetic spermaceti.

CETYL LACTATE: See *Cetyl Alcohol.*

CETYL MYRISTATE/CETETH-(#): See *Cetyl Alcohol.*

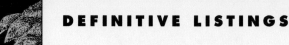

CETYL PALMITATE: See *Spermaceti* and *Cetyl Alcohol.*

CHOLESTERIN: Cholesterol. A steroid alcohol, especially in all animal fats and oils, nerve tissue, egg yolk and blood. Can be derived from lanolin (see). In cosmetics, eye creams, shampoos, etc. Alternatives: plant sources, synthetics.

CHOLESTEROL: See *Cholesterin.*

CHOLINE BITARTRATE: Lecithin. In all living organisms. Frequently obtained for commercial purposes from eggs and soybeans (when stated *soy lecithin*). Also from nerve tissue, blood, milk, corn. Choline bitartrate, the basic constituent of lecithin, is in many animal and plant tissues or prepared synthetically. Lecithin can be in eye creams, lipsticks, liquid powders, hand creams, lotions, soaps, shampoos, other cosmetics, candies, other foods and medicines.

CIVET: Obtained from the civet, a small mammal, by stimulating it, usually through torture. Civets are kept captive in cages in horrible conditions. Used in perfumes as a fixative.

COCHINEAL (E120): See *Carmine.*

COD LIVER OIL: Fish Liver Oil. Fish Livers. Used in lubricating creams and lotions, vitamins and supplements. In milk fortified with Vitamin D. Alternatives: vegetable oils, yeast extract ergosterol, sunshine.

COLLAGEN: A fibrous protein in vertebrates. Usually derived from animal tissue. In cosmetics. Can't affect the skin's own collagen. Alternatives: soy protein, almond oil, amla oil (from Indian tree's fruit).

CORTICO STEROID: Cortisone. Hormone from cattle liver. Widely used in medicine. Alternatives: synthetics.

CORTISONE: See *Cortico Steroid.*

CYSTEINE, L-FORM: Cystine. Two amino acids that can come from animals. Used in hair products and creams, in some bakery products and wound healing formulations. Alternatives: plant sources.

CYSTINE: See *Cysteine, L-Form.*

DNA/RNA: Deoxyribonucleic Acid. Ribonucleic Acid. Polypeptides. Obtained from slaughterhouse wastes. In all living cells. Used in many protein shampoos and cosmetics. Alternatives: plant cells.

DEOXYRIBONUCLEIC ACID: See *DNA/RNA.*

DEPANTHENOL: Panthenol. Vitamin B Complex Factor. Provitamin B5. Can come from animal or plant sources or synthetics. In shampoos, foods, supplements, emollients, etc.

DIGLYCERIDES: Monoglycerides. Glycerides. From animal fat. In margarines, cake mixes, confectionaries, foods, peanut butter, non-dairy coffee creamer, cosmetics, etc. Glycerin (see). Alternatives: vegetable monoglycerides and diglycerides, synthetics.

DOWN: Goose or duck insulating feathers. Often from slaughtered or cruelly exploited geese. Used in pillows and as an insulator in quilts, parkas and sleeping bags. Bad in cold, wet weather as it packs down. Alternatives: many polyester and man-made substitutes, superior in many ways; Kapok (silky fibers from the seeds of some tropical trees); milkweed seedpod fibers.

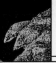

DUODENUM SUBSTANCES: From the digestive tracts of cattle and swine. In some vitamins and medicines. Alternatives: vegetarian vitamins, synthetics.

E120: See *Carmine*.

EGG ALBUMEN/ALBUMIN: See *Albumen*.

EGG PROTEIN: In shampoos, skin preparations, etc. Alternatives: plant proteins.

ELASTIN: Found in the neck ligaments and aorta of bovine. Similar to collagen. Can't affect the skin's own elasticity. Alternatives: synthetics, proteins from plant tissues.

ERGOSTEROL: See *Calciferol*.

ERGOCALCIFEROL: See *Calciferol*.

ESTRADIOL: Estrone. Estrogen. From cow ovaries and pregnant mares' urine. Considered a drug. Can have harmful systemic effects if used by children. Used for reproductive problems and in birth control pills. In creams and lotions. Has no effect in the creams as a "nourishing" factor and simple vegetable source creams are considered better. Alternatives: Oral contraceptives marketed today are usually based on synthetic steroids. Phytoestrogens (from plants) are being researched currently.

ESTROGEN: See *Estradiol*.

ESTRONE: See *Estradiol*.

FATTY ACIDS: Can be one or any mixture of liquid and solid acids, caprylic, myristic, oleic, palmitic, stearic, behenic. Used in bubble baths, lipsticks, soaps, detergents, cosmetics, shampoos, foods. Alternatives: vegetable-derived acids, soy lecithin, safflower oil, bitter almond oil, sunflower oil, etc.

FEATHERS: Down (see). Keratin (see). Generally from exploited and/or slaughtered birds. Can be used as ornaments in whole or can be ground up in shampoos, etc.

FISH LIVER(S): See *Cod Liver Oil.*

FISH LIVER OIL: See *Cod Liver Oil.*

FISH OIL: Marine Oil. From fish or marine mammals (including porpoises). Used in soap making, candles, lubricants, paints and as a shortening (especially in some margarines). (US regulations currently prohibit the use of ingredients derived from marine mammals.)

FISH SCALES: Used in shimmery makeups (eye, etc.). Garbage cans full of scales are sold to manufacturers. Alternatives: mica, rayon.

FLETAN OIL: Rare ingredient derived from fish liver that includes lecithin, Vitamin A and Vitamin D (see all).

FUR: Hopefully speaks for itself.

GELATIN: Gel. Protein obtained by boiling skin, tendons, ligaments or bones with water, from cattle and hogs. Used in shampoos, face masks, other cosmetics. Used as a thickener for fruit gelatins and puddings (Jello-brand desserts). In candies, marshmallows, cakes, ice cream, yogurts. On photographic film as a coat-

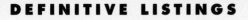

ing and in vitamins as capsules. Sometimes used to assist in "clearing" wines. Alternatives: algae and seaweed (carrageen/Irish Moss, algin, agar-agar, kelp); Gelozone, used in jellies, plastics, medicines, pectin from fruit, dextrins, locust bean gum and cotton gum. Marshmallows were originally made from the root of the marshmallow plant.

GEL: See *Gelatin*.

GLUTAMIC ACID: An amino acid found widely in plant and animal tissue. Used as food seasoning and as an antioxidant in cosmetics.

GLYCERIDES: See *Diglycerides*.

GLYCERIN: Glycerine. Glycerol. Polyglycerol. Polyethylene Glycol (PEG). A byproduct of soap manufacture (normally using animal fat). In cosmetics, foods, mouthwashes, toothpastes, soaps, ointments, medicines, lubricants, transmission and brake fluids, plastics. Alternatives: vegetable or vegetable glycerin, a byproduct of vegetable oil soap; derivatives of seaweed; petroleum.

GLYCERINE: See *Glycerin*.

GLYCEROL: See *Diglycerides*.

GOOSE INSULATING FEATHERS: See *Down*.

GUANINE: Pearl Essence. Obtained from scales of fish. Constituent of ribonucleic acid and deoxyribonucleic acid and is found in all animal and plant tissues. In shampoos, nail polish, other cosmetics. Alternatives: leguminous plants, synthetics.

HIDE GLUE: Same as gelatin but of a cruder, more impure form. Alternatives: dextrins and synthetic petrochemical-based adhesives.

HONEY: Food for bees, made by bees. Still a sugar, too concentrated for humans. Contains toxins harmful to humans. Can cause allergic reactions. In cosmetics, foods. Alternatives: maple syrup, date sugar, syrups made from grains.

HORSEHAIR AND OTHER ANIMAL HAIR: In some blankets mattresses, brushes, furniture, etc. Alternatives: vegetable and man-made fibers.

HYDROLYZED ANIMAL PROTEIN: In cosmetics, especially shampoos and hair treatments. Alternatives: soy protein, other vegetable proteins, amla oil (from an Indian tree's fruit).

HYDROLYZED MILK PROTEIN: Milk Protein. From cow's milk. In cosmetics, shampoos, moisturizers, conditioners, etc. Alternatives: soy protein, other plant proteins.

IMIDAZOLIDINYL UREA: See *Carbamide.*

INSULIN: From the pancreas of hogs and oxen. Used by millions of diabetics daily. Alternatives: synthetics, human insulin grown in a lab, diet when possible.

ISINGLASS: A form of gelatin prepared from the internal membranes of fish bladders. In foods and sometimes used in "clearing" wines and beers. Alternatives: bentonite clay, "Japanese isinglass" (see *Alternatives for Gelatin*). Isinglass is also a mineral, mica, used in cosmetics.

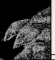
ISOPROPYL MYRISTATE: Myristate Acid. Myristyl. In most animal and vegetable fats. In butter acids. Used in shampoos, creams, cosmetics, food flavorings. Alternatives: nut butters, oil of lovage, coconut oil, extract from seed kernels of nutmeg, etc.

KERATIN: From the ground-up horns, hoofs, feathers, quills and hair of various creatures. In hair rinses, shampoos, permanent wave solutions. Alternatives: almond oil, soy protein, amla oil (from an Indian tree's fruit), rosemary, nettle. Rosemary and nettle give body and strand strength to hair.

L-FORM: See *Cysteine*.

L-LACTIC ACID: Lactic Acid (a by-product of the slaughter-house). Produced by the fermentation of lactose when milk sours or from sucrose and some other carbohydrates by the action of certain microorganisms. Can be found in blood and muscle tissue. In skin fresheners, adhesives, plasticizers, pharmaceuticals, sour milk, beer, sauerkraut, pickles and other food products made by bacterial fermentation. Used in foods and beverages as an acidulant, flavoring and preservative.

LACTIC ACID: See *L-Lactic Acid*.

LACTOSE: Milk Sugar. Milk of mammals. In eye lotions, foods, tablets, cosmetics, baked goods, medicines, shampoos. Alternatives: plant milk sugars.

LANOLIN: Lanolin Acid. Lanolin Alcohols (Sterol, Triterpene Alcohol, Aliphatic Alcohol). Wool Fat. Laneth-5, -10, etc. Lanogene. Lanosterol. Isopropyl Lanolate. A product of the oil glands of sheep, extracted from their wool (see). In many skin care products and cosmetics and in medicines. Some cosmetic companies won't use it because it commonly causes allergic contact skin rashes, and also they consider it to be a cheap filler. Vegetable sources are thought to be better moisturizers; lanolin is too greasy, waterproof and sealing – skin can't breathe.

LANOLIN ACID: See *Lanolin*.

LANOLIN ALCOHOLS: See *Lanolin*.

LANOSTEROL: See *Lanolin*.

LARD: Fat from hog abdomens. In shaving creams, soaps, cosmetics, baked goods and other foods. Hard to digest. Alternatives: vegetable fats or oils.

LEATHER: Suede. Calfskin. Sheepskin. Alligator. Kid. Euphemism for animal skin. The use of and sale of it subsidizes the meat industry. Used to make wallets, handbags, belts, furniture, and car upholstery, shoes, coats, etc. Alternatives: natural materials such as cotton and canvas. Also man-made materials such as nylon and vinyl.

LECITHIN: See *Choline Bitartrate*.

LINOLEIC ACID: An essential fatty acid (see). In cosmetics, vitamins.

LIPASE: Enzyme from the stomachs and tongue glands of calves, kids and lambs. Probably in some vitamins. Alternatives: vegetable enzymes.

LIPOIDS/LIPIDS: Fat and fat-like substances that occur in animals and plants.

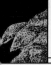

LUNA SPONGE: Sea Sponge. A plant-like animal that lives in the sea and is becoming scarce. Alternatives: man-made sponges.

MARINE OIL: See *Fish Oil*.

METHIONINE: An essential amino acid found in various proteins. Used as a texturizer in creams.

MILK OF MAMMALS: If this isn't already obvious, see *Lactose*.

MILK PROTEIN: Hydrolyzed Milk Protein (see). From cow's milk. In cosmetics, shampoos, moisturizers, conditioners, etc. Alternatives: soy protein, other plant proteins.

MILK SUGAR: See *Lactose*.

MINK OIL: From minks. In cosmetics, creams, etc. Alternatives: vegetable oils and emollients (i.e. avocado, almond oil, jojoba).

MONOGLYCERIDES: See *Diglycerides*.

MUSK: Obtained from the genitals of the Northern Asian small hornless deer. In perfumes and food flavorings. Can cause allergic reactions. Alternatives: labdanum (oil which comes from various rockrose shrubs) — no known toxicity. Other plants have a musky scent also.

MYRISTATE ACID: See *Isopropyl Myristate*.

MYRISTYL: See *Isopropyl Myristate*.

NATURAL FLAVOR: Natural Flavoring. Natural Source. Can mean animal, vegetable or mineral source. Most often in the health

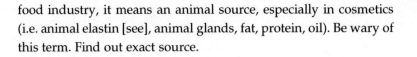

food industry, it means an animal source, especially in cosmetics (i.e. animal elastin [see], animal glands, fat, protein, oil). Be wary of this term. Find out exact source.

NATURAL SOURCE: See *Natural Flavor*.

NUCLEIC ACID: In the nucleus of all living cells. Used in cosmetics, shampoos, conditioners, vitamins, supplements, etc. Alternatives: plant sources.

OCTYL DODECANOL: Mixture of solid waxy alcohols. Primarily from stearyl alcohol (see).

OLEAN®: Olestra®. A man-made fat substitute that contains fatty acids (see). Originally planned to market as a drug. Depletes body of, and prevents absorption of vitamins. In some potato chips and other fried foods. Alternatives: plant sources. (See pg. 11 for more information)

OLEIC ACID: Oleth-2, -3, -20, etc. Oleyl Alcohol. Oleamine. Oleyl Betaine. Obtained from various animal and vegetable fats and oils. Is usually obtained commercially from inedible tallow (see), sometimes synthesized from petroleum. In foods, soft soaps, bar soaps, permanent wave solutions, shampoos, creams, nail polish, lipsticks, liquid makeups, and many other skin preparations. Alternatives: coconut oil (see alternatives for Animal Oils and Fats).

OLESTRA®: See *Olean®*.

OLETH-2, -3, -20, ETC./OLEYL ALCOHOL/ OLEAMINE/OLEYL BETAINE: See *Oleic Acid*.

OLYL ALCOHOL/BETAINE: See *Oleic Acid*.

OX BILE: Oxgall. From castrated bovines. In creams.

OXGALL: See *Ox Bile*.

PALMITATE: Palmitic Acid. Fatty Acids (see). From fats, oils, mixed with stearic acid (see). Occurs in many animal fats and plant oils. In shampoos, shaving soaps, creams. Alternatives: palm oil and other vegetable source.

PALMITIC ACID: See *Palmitate*.

PANTHENOL: See *Depanthenol*.

PEARL ESSENCE: See *Guanine*.

PEPSIN: Obtained from the stomachs of hogs. A clotting agent. In some cheeses and vitamins. Same uses and alternatives as rennet (see).

PLACENTA: See *Afterbirth*.

PLACENTA POLYPEPTIDES PROTEIN: See *Afterbirth*.

POLYGLYCEROL: See *Glycerin*.

POLYPEPTIDES: See *DNA/RNA*.

POLYPEPTIDES PROTEIN: See *Afterbirth*.

POLYSORBATES: Derivatives of fatty acids (see). In cosmetics, foods.

POLYETHYLENE GLYCEROL/PEG: See *Glycerin*.

PRISTANE: Obtained from the liver oil of sharks and from whale ambergris (see). See *Squalene*. Used as a lubricant and anti-corrosive agent. In cosmetics. (US regulations currently prohibit the use of ingredients derived from marine mammals. Alternatives: plant oils, synthetics.)

PROGESTERONE: A steroid hormone (see) used in face creams. Can have adverse systemic effects. Alternatives: synthetics.

PROPOLIS: A resinous substance collected from various plants by bees and used in the construction of their hives. In toothpastes, shampoos, deodorants, supplements, etc.

PROVITAMIN A: See *Beta Carotene*.

PROVITAMIN B5: See *Depanthenol*.

QUATERNIUM 27: Tallow (see). Stearamide. Stearate. Stearic Acid. Stearin. Fat from cows, sheep, etc. (could be dogs and cats from shelters). Most often refers to a fatty substance taken from the stomachs of pigs. Can be harsh, irritating. Used in cosmetics, soaps, lubricants, candles, hairsprays, conditioners, deodorants, creams. Alternatives: can be found in many vegetable fats (i.e. coconut).

RENNET: Rennin. From calves' stomachs. Used in cheesemaking, rennet custard (junket) and in many coagulated dairy products. Alternatives: microbial coagulating agents, bacteria culture, lemon juice.

RENNIN: See *Rennet*.

RETINOL: See *Acetate*.

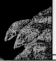

RIBONUCLEIC ACID: See *DNA/RNA*.

RNA/DNA: See *DNA/RNA*.

ROYAL JELLY: Secretion of the throat glands of the honeybee workers that is fed to the larvae in a colony and to all queens' larvae. No proven value in cosmetic preparations. Alternatives: aloe vera, comfrey, other plant derivatives.

SABLE BRUSHES: From the fur of sables (weasel-like mammals). Used to make cosmetic brushes. Alternatives: synthetic furs and fibers.

SEA SPONGE: See *Luna Sponge*.

SEA TURTLE OIL: Turtle Oil. From the muscles and genitals of giant sea turtles. In soaps, skin creams, nail creams, other cosmetics. Alternatives: vegetable emollients. See alternatives for *Animal Oils and Fats*.

SHEEPSKIN: See *Leather*.

SHELLAC: Obtained from the bodies of the female scale insect Tachardia lacca. Shellac is used as varnish, as a coating on wood and plaster, in electrical insulation, and in sealing wax.

SILK: Shiny fiber made by silkworms to form their cocoons. Boiled or roasted in their cocoons to get the silk. Used in cloth and silk screening. Alternatives: milkweed seed pod fibers, nylon, silk-cotton tree and ceiba tree filaments (kapok), rayon, man-made silks. Other fine cloth can be and is used for silk screening. Taffeta can be made from silk or nylon.

SILK POWDER: Obtained from the secretion of the silkworm. Used as a coloring agent in face powders, soaps, etc. Causes severe allergic reactions; systemic reactions if inhaled or ingested.

SNAILS: Crushed. In some cosmetics.

SPERMACETI: Cetyl Palmitate. Sperm Oil. Waxy oil derived from the sperm whale's head or from dolphins. In skin creams, ointments, shampoos, candles, many margarines. Used in the leather industry. May become rancid and cause irritations. (US regulations currently prohibit the use of ingredients derived from marine mammals.) Alternatives: synthetic spermaceti, jojoba oil and other vegetable emollients.

SPERM OIL: See *Spermaceti*.

SQUALANE: Squalene (see). Obtained from shark liver oil. Lubricant and perfume fixative. Alternatives: synthetics.

SQUALENE: Squalane (see). Obtained from shark liver oil or vegetable oil. An emollient from a "natural source" (see). A precursor of cholesterol in biosynthesis. In cosmetics, moisturizers, hair dyes. Alternatives: vegetable emollients (olive oil, wheat germ oil, rice bran oil, etc.).

STEARAMIDE/STEARATE/STEARIN: See *Quaternium 27*.

STEARIC ACID: See *Quaternium 27*.

STEARYL ALCOHOL: Stenol. A mixture of solid alcohols; can be prepared from sperm whale oil. In medicines, creams, rinses, shampoos, etc. (US regulations currently prohibit the use of ingredients derived from marine mammals.) Alternatives: plant tissues, synthetics.

STENOL: See *Stearyl Alcohol.*

STEROID: Sterol. From various animal glands or from plant tissues. Steroids include sterols. Sterols are alcohols from animals or plants (i.e. cholesterol). Used in hormone preparations. In creams, lotions, hair conditioners, fragrances, etc. Alternatives: plant tissues, synthetics.

STEROL: See *Steroid.*

SUEDE: See *Leather.*

TALLOW: Tallowate. Tallow Fatty Alcohol. Stearic Acid (see). Rendered beef or sheep fat. May cause eczema and blackheads. In wax paper, crayons, margarines, paints, rubber, lubricants, candles, soaps, shampoos, lipsticks, shaving creams, other cosmetics. Alternatives: vegetable tallow (animal tallow usually used commercially), Japan tallow, paraffin, ceresin. See alternatives for *Beeswax.*

TALLOWATE: See *Tallow.*

TALLOW FATTY ALCOHOL: See *Tallow.*

TURTLE OIL: See *Sea Turtle Oil.*

UREA: See *Carbamide.*

URIC ACID: See *Carbamide.*

VITAMIN A: Retinol. Acetate (see) and Palmitate. (See *Palmitic Acid.*)

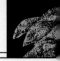

VITAMIN B COMPLEX FACTOR: Provitamin B5. Depanthenol (see). Panthenol.

VITAMIN B FACTOR: See *Biotin.*

VITAMIN B12: Usually from an animal source. Some vegetarian B12 fortified yeasts and analogs available. Some vegetarian B12 vitamins are in a stomach base. Plant algae discovered containing B12, now in supplement form (spirulina). Also, B12 is produced in a healthy body.

VITAMIN D: See *Calciferol.*

VITAMIN H: See *Biotin.*

VITAMINS, OTHER: (Choline, Biotin [see], Inositol, Riboflavin, etc.). Many other vitamins can come from animal sources. Alternatives: vegetarian vitamins, plant and mineral sources.

WHEY: From milk. Usually in cakes, cookies, candies, cheese. Alternatives: soybean whey.

WOOL: From sheep (in the US, mostly from slaughtered ones). Used in clothing, including blends. Ram lambs and old "wool" sheep are slaughtered for their meat and last shearing. Sheep are transported without food or water in extreme heat and cold. Legs are broken, eyes injured, etc. Sheep are bred to be unnaturally woolly. Inferior sheep are killed. Shearing DOES hurt the sheep. They are pinned down violently, sheared roughly. Their skin is cut up. Every year, hundreds of thousands of shorn sheep die from exposure to cold. Natural predators of sheep (wolves, coyotes, eagles, etc.) are poisoned, trapped and shot. In the US, overgrazing by cattle and sheep is turning more than 150 million acres of land into desert. "Natural" wool raising uses enormous amounts of resources and energy (to breed, raise, feed, shear, transport and slaughter the sheep). Many people are allergic to wool. Alternatives: cotton, cotton flannel, linen, man made fibers.

WOOL FAT: See *Lanolin*.

INGREDIENTS DERIVED FROM ANIMALS

A

Acetate
Acetylated Hydrogenated Lard Glyceride
Acetylated Lanolin
Acetylated Lanolin Alcohol
Acetylated Lanolin Ricinoleate
Acetylated Tallow
Afterbirth
Adrenaline
Albumen
Albumin
Aldioxa
Aliphatic Alcohol
Allantoin
Alpha-Hydroxy Acids
Ambergris
Amerachol™
Amino Acids
Aminosuccinate Acid; DL and L Forms
Ammonium Hydrolyzed Protein
Amniotic Fluid
AMPD Isoteric Hydrolyzed Animal Protein
Amylase
Angora
Animal Bones
Animal Collagen Amino Acids
Animal Keratin Amino Acids
Animal Oils & Fats
Animal Protein Derivative

Animal Tissue Extract – Epiderm Oil R
Arachidonic Acid
Arachidyl Proprionate
Aspartic Acid
Aspic

B

Batyl Alcohol
Batyl Isostearate
Bee Products
Bee Pollen
Beeswax
Benzoic Acid
Benzyltrimonium Hydrolyzed Animal Protein
Biotin
Blood
Boar Bristles
Bone Ash
Bone Black
Boneblack
Bone Charcoal
Bone Earth
Bonemeal
Brain Extract
Buttermilk

C

C30-46 Piscine Oil
Calciferol
Calfskin Extract
Cantharides Tincture – Spanish Fly

Carbamide

Carmine – Cochineal

Carminic Acid – Natural Red No. 4

Caprylic Acid

Caprylic Triglyceride

Carbamide

Carmine

Carminic Acid

Carotene

Casein

Cashmere

Castor – Castoreum (not Castor Oil)

Catgut

Catharidin

Cera Flava

Cerebrosides

Ceteth-2 – Polyethylene (2) Cetyl Ether

Ceteth-2, -4, -6, -10, -30

Cetyl Alcohol

Cetyl Lactate

Cetyl Myristate

Cetyl Palmitate

Chitosan

Cholesterin

Cholesterol

Choleth-24

Choline Bitartrate

Civet

Cochineal

Cod-Liver Oil

Collagen

Cortico Steroid
Cortisone
Cysteine, L-Form
Cystine (or Cysteine)

D

Dea-Oleth-10 Phosphate
Deoxyribonucleic Acid
Depanthenol
Desamido Animal Collagen
Desamidocollagen
Dicapryloyl Cystine
Diethylene Tricaseinamide
Diglycerides
Dihydrocholesterol
Dihydrocholesterol Octyledecanoate
Dihydrocholeth-15
Dihydrocholeth-30
Dihydrogenated Tallow Benzylmoniumchloride
Dihydrogenated Tallow Methylamine
Dihydrogenated Tallow Phthalate
Dihydroxyethyl Tallow Amine Oxide
Dimethyl Hydrogenated Tallowamine
Dimethyl Stearamine
Dimethyl Tallowamine
Disodium Hydrogenated TallowGlutamate
Disodium Tallamido Mea-Sulfosuccinate
Disodium Tallowaminodipropionate
Ditallowdimonium Chloride
Down
Dried Buttermilk

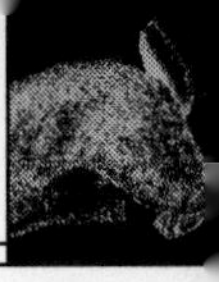

Dried Egg Yolk
Duodenum Substances

E

E120
E542
Edible Bone Phosphate
Egg
Egg Albumen
Egg Albumin
Egg Oil
Egg Powder
Egg Protein
Egg Yolk
Egg Yolk Extract
Elastin
Embryo Extract
Emu Oil
Ergosterol
Estradiol
Estradiol Benzoate
Estrogen
Estrone
Ethyl Arachidonate
Ethyl Ester of Hydrolyzed Animal Protein
Ethyl Morrhuate – Lipineate
Ethylene Dehydrogenated Tallowamide

F

Fatty Acids
Feathers

Fish Glycerides
Fish Liver Oil
Fish Oil
Fletan Oil
Fur

G

Gelatin (not Gel)
Glucose Tyrosinase
Glucuronic Acid
Glutamic Acid
Glycreth-26
Glycerides
Glycerin
Glycerol
Glyceryl Lanolate
Glycogen
Guanine – Pearl Essence

H

Heptylundecanol
Hide Glue
Honey
Horsehair
Human Placental Protein
Human Umbilical Extract
Hyaluronic Acid
Hydrocortisone
Hydrogenated Animal Glyceride
Hydrogenated Ditallow Amine
Hydrogenated Honey
Hydrogenated Laneth-5, -20, -25
Hydrogenated Lanolin
Hydrogenated Lanolin Alcohol

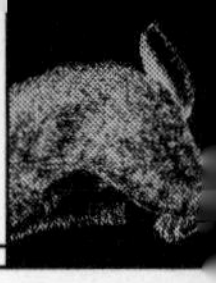

Hydrogenated Lard Glyceride
Hydrogenated Shark-Liver Oil
Hydrogenated Tallow Acid
Hydrogenated Tallow Betaine
Hydrogenated Tallow Glyceride
Hydrolyzed Animal Elastin
Hydrolyzed Animal Keratin
Hydrolyzed Animal Protein
Hydrolyzed Casein
Hydrolyzed Elastin
Hydrolyzed Human Placental Protein
Hydrolyzed Keratin
Hydrolyzed Silk
Hydroxylated Lanolin

I

Imidazolidinyl Urea
Insulin
Isinglass
Isobutylated Lanolin
Isopropyl Lanolate
Isopropyl Myristate
Isopropyl TallowateIsopropyl Lanolate
Isostearic Hydrolyzed Animal Protein
Isostearoyl Hydrolyzed Animal Protein

K

Keratin
Keratin Amino Acids

L

Lactic Acid
Lactic Yeasts
Lactose – Milk Sugar

Laneth-5 through -40

Laneth-9 and -10 Acetate

Lanogene

Lanolin – Wool Fat; Wool Wax

Lanolin Acid

Lanolin Alcohols – Sterols; Triterpene Alcohols; Aliphatic
   Alcohols

Lanolin Linoleate

Lanolin Oil

Lanolin Ricinoleate

Lanolin Wax

Lanoinamide DEA

Lanosteral

Lard

Lard Glyceride

Lauroyl Hydrolyzed Animal Protein

Leather

Lecithin

Leucine

L-Lactic Acid

Linoleic Acid

Lipace

Lipoids

Lipids

Liver Extract

Luna Sponge

Lysine

M

Magnesium Lanolate

Magnesium Tallowate

Mammarian Extract
Marine Oil
Mayonnaise
MEA-Hydrolyzed Animal Protein
Menhaden Oil – Pogy Oil; Mossbunker Oil
Methionine
Milk
Milk Protein
Mink Oil
Minkamidopropyl Diethylamine
Monoglycerides
Muscle Extract
Musk
Musk Ambrette
Myristic Acid
Myristoyl
Myristoyl Hydrolyzed Animal Protein

N

Neat's-Foot Oil
Nucleic Acid

O

Ocenol
Octyl Dodecanol
Olean®
Oleamidopropyl Dimethylamine Hydrolyzed Animal Protein
Oleic Acid
Oleostearine
Oleoyl Hydrolyzed Animal Protein
Olestra®

Oleth-2, and 3

Oleth-5, and 10

Oleth-25 and 50

Oleyl Alcohol

Oleyl Arachidate

Oleyl Betatine

Oleyl Imidazoline

Oleyl Lanolate

Ovarian Extract

Ox Bile

P

Palmitate

Palmitic Acid

Palmitoyl Hydrolyzed Animal Protein

Palmitoyl Hydrolyzed Milk Protein

Panthenol

PEG-28 Glyceryl Tallowate

PEG-8 Hydrogenated Fish Glycerides

PEG-5 through -70 Hydrogenated Lanolin

PEG-13 Hydrogenated Tallow Amide

PEG-5 to -20 Lanolate

PEG-5 through -100 Lanolin

PEG-75 Lanolin Oil and Wax

PEG-2 Milk Solids

PEG-6, -8, -20 Sorbitan Beeswax

PEG-40, -75, or -80 Sorbitan Lanolate

PEG-3, -10, or -15 Tallow Aminopropylamine

PEG-15 Tallow Polyamine

PEG-20 Tallowate

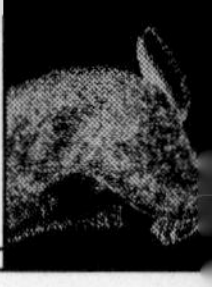

Pentahydrosqualene

Pepsin

Perhydrosqualene

Pigskin Extract

Placenta

Placenta Polypeptides Protein

Placental Enzymes, Lipids and Proteins

Placental Extract

Placental Protein

Polyglycerol

Polyglyceryl-2 Lanolin Alcohol Ether

Polypeptide(s)

Polysorbate(s)

Polyethylene Glycol (PEG)

Potassium Caseinate

Potassium Tallowate

Potassium Undecylenoyl Hydrolyzed Animal Protein

PPG-12-PEG-50 Lanolin

PPG-2, -5, -10. -20, -30 Lanolin Alcohol Ethers

PPG-30 Lanolin Ether

Pregnenolone Acetate

Pristane

Progesterone

Propolis

Purcelline Oil Syn

R

Royal jelly

Rennin

Rennet

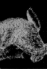

Resinous Glaze
Ribonucleic Acid
RNA/DNA

S

Sable Brushes
Saccharide Hydrolysate
Saccharide Isomerate
Sea Turtle Oil
Serum Albumin
Serum Proteins
Shark-Liver Oil
Shellac
Shellac Wax
Silk
Silk Amino Acids
Silk Powder
Snail(s)
Sodium Caseinate
Sodium Chondroitin Sulfate
Sodium Coco-Hydrolyzed Animal Protein
Sodium Hydrogenated Tallow Glutamate
Sodium Laneth Sulfate
Sodium Methyl Oleoyl Taurate
Sodium n-Methyl-n-Oleyl Taurate
Sodium Soy Hydrolyzed Animal Protein
Sodium Tallow Sulfate
Sodium Tallowate
Sodium / TEA-Lauroyl Hydrolyzed Animal Protein
Sodium / TEA-Undecylenoyl Hydrolyzed Animal Protein
Sodium Undecylenate

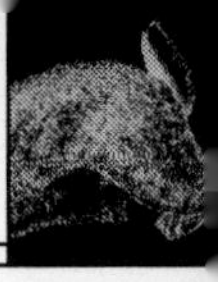

Soluble (Animal) Collagen
Soy Hydroxyethyl Imidazoline
Spermaceti
Sperm Oil
Spleen Extract
Squalane
Squalene
Stearamide
Stearamine Oxide
Stearic Acid
Stearone
Stearyl Alcohol – Stenol
Stearyldimethyl Amine
Stearyl Imidazoline
Sterols

T

Tallow
Tallow Acid
Tallow Amide
Tallow Aminopropylamine Oxide
Tallow Amine
Tallow Amine Oxide
Tallow Fatty Alcohol
Tallow Glycerides
Tallow Hydroxyethyl Imidazoline
Tallow Imidazoline
Tallowate
Tallowmide DEA and MEA
Tallowmidopropyl Hydroxysultaine
Tallowminopropylamine

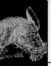
Tallowmphoacete
Talloweth-6
Tallow Trimonium Chloride – Tallow
Tea-Abietoyl Hydrolyzed Animal Protein
Tea-Coco Hydrolyzed Animal Protein
Tea-Lauroyl Animal Collagen Amino Acids
Tea-Lauroyl Animal Keratin Amino Acids
Tea-Myristol Hydrolyzed Animal Protein
Tea-Undecylenoyl Hydrolyzed Animal Protein
Testicular Extract
Threonine
Triethonium Hydrolyzed Animal Protein Ethosulfate
Trilaneth-4 Phosphate
Triterpine Alcohols
Turtle Oil

U

Urea
Uric Acid

W

Whey
Wood Fat
Wool
Wool Wax Alcohols

Y

Yogurt

Z

Zinc Hydrolyzed Animal Protein

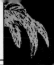

With the growing number of microbreweries and the number of corporate breweries introducing new beers that pose as microbrews, a complete list of beers that are suitable for vegans would have to be updated daily. In this chapter we have attempted to note more popular beers. We have also attempted to note which breweries don't typically use animal products in their brewing process. As always, common sense should prevail. If one of the brands listed here releases a honey porter after this book goes to print, it is obviously not vegan. We have also tried to provide a lot of general information on the brewing of beers to assist in making an educated guess. If all else fails, the best means of finding out if a particular beer is vegan is to contact the manufacturer.

Since the last edition, cider has become an integral part of US drinking culture, so we've tried to provide as much information as we could find on the ever-confusing world of cider. Unfortunately the myth is not true that vegan alcoholic beverages give you less of a hangover.

VEGAN BEERS

Vegetarian Times and the *Bay Vegan* found that animal products aren't generally used in beer brewing in the US. Gelatin used to be widely used in beer manufacturing in the US, but most major brewing companies haven't included gelatin in beer for some time.

Those on the following list are all acceptable for vegetarians and vegans.

BITTERS, ETC.

Alloa Light..keg
Alloa 70/Special ....keg, can & bottle
Alloa 80/Export ....keg, can & bottle
Alloa Stout..bottle

Batemans IPA ....bottle
Batemans Nut Brown..bottle
Batemans; XXXB ....bottle
Batemans Victory Ale ....bottle
Batemans Dark Mild ....bottle
Batemans GB Bitter ....bottle
Burtonwood Bitter ....keg & can
Burtonwood Mild..keg
Burtonwood Pale Mild ....keg
Burtonwood Top Hat Ale ....keg
Drybrough Heavy ....keg
Drybrough Best Scotch ....bottle
Felinfoel Bitter..keg & can
Felinfoel Double Dragon Bitter................keg & can
Fuller's London Pride....................keg, can & bottle
Fuller's Chiswick Bitter ....keg & can
Fuller's Mild ....keg
Fuller's ESB Export...bottle
Fuller's Pale Ale ....bottle
Fuller's Brown Ale ....bottle
Fullers LA ....bottle
Gale's Southdown Bitter ....keg
Gale's Best Bitter...keg
Gale's 777 Mild ....keg
Gale's Prize Old Ale ....bottle
Gale's Pale Ale ....bottle
Gale's HSB ....can
Golden Promise Organic Beer ....bottle
Hall & Woodhouse BXB Bitter...........................keg
H & W Malthouse Bitter ....keg
H & W Oasthouse Bitter ....can
H & W Badger Country Bitter ....can
H & W Tanglefoot Bitter ....can
Morrells Friars Bitter ....keg

Morrells Castle Ale..bottle
Morrells Light Ale ....bottle
Morrells College Ale ....bottle
Morrells Brewery Gate Bitter ....can
Redruth Brewery Bitter.....................................can
Redruth Brewery Mile Ale ....can
Redruth Aston Manor Bitter...............................can
Redruth Gold Cap Bitter ....can
Redruth Brewster Bitter....................................can
Redruth John Davey Bitter ....keg & can
Robinson's Best Bitter ....can
Ross Brewery Hartcliffe Bitter ....bottle
Ross Brewery Clifton Dark Ale ....bottle
Ross Brewery Saxon Ale ....bottle
Sainsburys Premium Ale...................................bottle
Sam Smiths Old Brewery......................keg & can
Sam Smiths Sovereign Best....................................keg
Sam Smiths Tadcaster Bitter..............................keg
Sam Smiths 4X Best Mild ....keg
Sam Smiths Dark Mild Ale.................................keg
Sam Smiths OB Strong Brown ....bottle
Sam Smiths OB Strong Pale ....bottle
Sam Smiths Pale Ale ....bottle
Sam Smiths Light Ale ....bottle
Sam Smiths Nut Brown....................................bottle
Sam Smiths Strong Golden ....bottle

LOW ALCOHOL, N/A

AyingerBrau Low Alcohol ....keg & bottle
Clausen..bottle
Greene King Lowes ....bottle
Marston's Low "C" ....keg & bottle
Wheelwright Low Alcohol ....keg & bottle

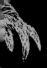

Wyvern Low Alcoholic ....bottle
Sharp's...can & bottle
Kingsbury...can & bottle
O'Douls Premium Non-Alcoholic Brew ....can & bottle

LAGERS

Aston Manor Lager ....can
AyingerBrau ....keg
AyingerBrau D. Pils ....keg & bottle
AyingerBrau Very Strong ....bottle
Brewster Lager ....can
Budweiser ....keg, can & bottle
Burtonwood Dagen ....can
Cornish Pilsner Lager ....can
Henri Funck...bottle
Grolsch ....keg, can & bottle
Guapa Lager ....bottle
Hall & Woodhouse Hectors ....can
H & W Forum ....can
H & W Compass..can
H & W Skona ....can
H & W Royal Hofbrau...can
Harp ....keg, can & bottle
Harp Extra...keg
Heineken Export............................keg, can & bottle
Heineken ....keg, can & bottle
Holsten Pils ....can & bottle
Knight's...can & bottle
Labatt's...keg
Lincoln Green Organic ....can
Lowenbrau Strong ....keg
Mousel ....bottle
Norseman ....can

Pinkus Special Organic ....bottle
Prinz Strong ....keg
Redruth Brewery Pilsner.......................................can
Sam Smiths Natural Lager...................can & bottle
Scorpion Dry ....can & bottle
Skol ....keg, can & bottle
Tennent's Gold Bier ....bottle
TQ Lager ....bottle
Tuborg Gold ....keg, can & bottle

US DOMESTICS AND/OR BOTTLED IN THE US

In the January/February 1995 issue of Animal Times—PETA's bimonthly magazine—there is a list of "cruelty-free beers" that states "The following brewing companies have assured PETA in writing that all their various beers are made without animal-derived ingredients, additives, or processing agents." We have researched and expanded their existing list here.

Anchor Steam ....keg & bottle
Anderson Valley ....keg & bottle
Anheuser-Busch ....keg, can & bottle
Barley's ....keg, can & bottle
Beach...keg, can & bottle
Beck's ....keg, can & bottle
Big Dog's Hospitality Group ....keg, can & bottle
Blue Ridge ....keg, can & bottle
Brick ....keg, can & bottle
Carlsberg-Tetley ....keg, can & bottle
Columbus..bottle
Courage ....keg, can & bottle
Dallas County ....keg, can & bottle
Dempsey's ....keg, can & bottle
Deschutes...keg, can & bottle

Dock Street.....................................keg, can & bottle
Dubuque ....keg, can & bottle
Eddie McStiff's ....keg, can & bottle
Fremont ....keg, can & bottle
Fullers...keg, can & bottle
Golden Pacific ....keg, can. & bottle
Grant's Yakima ....keg, can & bottle
Greene King....................................keg, can & bottle
Grolsch ....keg, can & bottle
G. Heileman....................................keg, can & bottle
Irons ....keg, can & bottle
James Page......................................keg, can & bottle
Jones Street ....keg, can & bottle
Lagunitas ....keg & botlle
Lakefront ....keg, can & bottle
Latrobe (Rolling Rock)...................keg, can & bottle
Les Brasseurs du Nord ....keg, can & bottle
Lost Coast ....keg, can & bottle
Mad River ....keg, can & bottle
Manhattan Beach ....keg, can & bottle
Masters Brewpub & Brasserie ....keg, can & bottle
Miller ....keg, can & bottle
Miracle ....keg, can & bottle
Nelson...keg, can & bottle
Nevada City....................................keg, can & bottle
North Coast ....keg, can & bottle
Nouveaux Brasseurs-Bar L'Inox ....keg, can & bottle
Odell..keg, can & bottle
Onalaska...keg, can & bottle
Oranjeboom ....keg, can & bottle
Otter Creek ....keg, can & bottle
Otto Brothers' ....keg, can & bottle
Pacific Hop Exchange ....keg, can & bottle
Pennsylvania ....keg, can & bottle

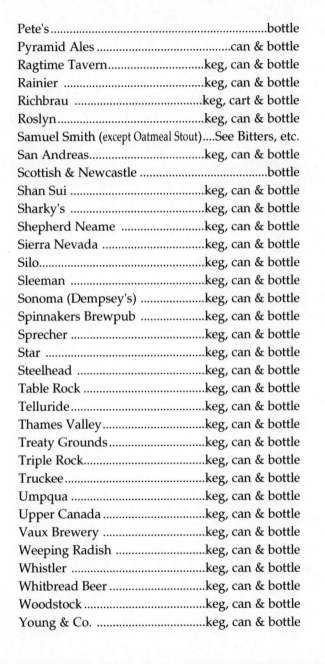

Pete's ....bottle
Pyramid Ales ....can & bottle
Ragtime Tavern...............................keg, can & bottle
Rainier ....keg, can & bottle
Richbrau ....keg, cart & bottle
Roslyn..keg, can & bottle
Samuel Smith (except Oatmeal Stout)....See Bitters, etc.
San Andreas....................................keg, can & bottle
Scottish & Newcastle ....bottle
Shan Sui ....keg, can & bottle
Sharky's ....keg, can & bottle
Shepherd Neame ....keg, can & bottle
Sierra Nevada ....keg, can & bottle
Silo..keg, can & bottle
Sleeman ....keg, can & bottle
Sonoma (Dempsey's) ....keg, can & bottle
Spinnakers Brewpub ....keg, can & bottle
Sprecher ....keg, can & bottle
Star ....keg, can & bottle
Steelhead ....keg, can & bottle
Table Rock ....keg, can & bottle
Telluride...keg, can & bottle
Thames Valley................................keg, can & bottle
Treaty Grounds..............................keg, can & bottle
Triple Rock......................................keg, can & bottle
Truckee...keg, can & bottle
Umpqua ....keg, can & bottle
Upper Canada ....keg, can & bottle
Vaux Brewery ....keg, can & bottle
Weeping Radish ....keg, can & bottle
Whistler ....keg, can & bottle
Whitbread Beer ....keg, can & bottle
Woodstock ....keg, can & bottle
Young & Co. ....keg, can & bottle

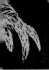

Most German beers are winners, because all are vegan. Bavarian purity laws limit them to four ingredients only: water, grain, hops and yeast.

Also: "Among the breweries making vegan nonalcoholic beer are Miller (Sharp's), Heileman (Kingsbury), and Anheuser-Busch (O'Doul's Premium Non-Alcoholic Brew)."

VEGAN WINES

Unfortunately many wines available in shops may have isinglass, gelatin, egg albumen (from battery eggs), chitin or even ox blood added as fining agents. Organic wines are much more likely to be vegetarian.

OUTSIDE OF THE U.S.

The use of animal-derived products in the production of alcoholic beverages outside of the U.S. is fairly widespread — not because alternatives do not exist, but because they always have been used and there is little demand from the consumer for an alternative.

The main obstacle when trying to judge the acceptability to vegetarians of any given product is a clause in the 1984 Food Labeling Regulations (UK) which excludes from the 1984 Food Act all drinks with an alcohol content exceeding 1.2% by volume (ABV), leaving only very low or non-alcoholic beers, wines and ciders being required to list all ingredients.

The main appearance of animal-derived products is in the fining or clearing process, though some others may be used as colorants or anti-foaming agents.

It must be pointed out that alcohol is routinely tested on thousands of animals each year. However, this is not usually done directly by any individual company.

BEER: Cask-conditioned ales need fining to clear the material (especially the yeast) held in suspension in the liquid. This is invariably done by adding isinglass, derived from the swim bladders of certain tropical fish, especially the Chinese sturgeon, which acts as a falling suspension. If you were to hold a pint of real ale up to the light and see cloudy lumps swirling around that would suggest that the cask had been recently disturbed and the isinglass shaken up from the bottom. Naturally bottled conditioned beers will not always have been treated with isinglass. Keg beers and Lagers are pasteurized and usually passed through Chill Filters, as are canned beers and some bottled beers. However, a considerable number of breweries still use isinglass to clear their pasteurized beers, though sometimes only to rescue selected batches which are considered too hazy. Also occasionally the sometimes animal-derived additive Glyceryl Monostearate is used in place of 900 Dimethylpolysiloxane as a foam-control agent in the production of keg beers.

It is sometimes possible to buy barrels of cask-conditioned beer from a brewery before it has been fined. The beer would then have to be left for a considerable time to stand before consumption. To our knowledge, only one pub in England sells unfined real ale on draught: The Cumberland Arms in Byker, Newcastle on Tyne.

Please refer to the list in this chapter for acceptable beers for vegans.

CIDER: Most of the main brands of cider will have been fined using gelatin. Scrumpy type ciders are less likely to have been fined (see the Cider section of this chapter).

WINE: With wine, it is again in the fining process that animal-derived ingredients make an appearance. Finings can be isinglass, gelatin, egg albumen, modified casein (from milk), chitin (derived from the shells of crabs or lobsters) or ox blood (rarely used today). But alternatives do exist in the form of bentonite, kieselguhr, kaolin and silica gel or solution. Also newer methods such as centrifuging and filtering are becoming more popular. The majority of organic wines do not use animal-derived finings – but some do. Thorson's Organic Wine Guide by Jerry Lockspeiser and Jackie Gear, published in 1991, lists those wines which are suitable. You might like to note that the Wine Development Board claim that the fining agents are removed at the end of the process with the possible exception of very minute quantities.

SPIRITS: Most spirits appear to be acceptable to vegetarians, with the possible exception of Malt Whisky, some blended whiskies and Spanish Brandies that have been conditioned in casks that had previously held sherry that may have been treated with animal-derived finings (brandy itself is not produced from wine that has undergone any fining processes). Also some imported vodkas may have been passed through a bone charcoal filter.

FORTIFIED WINES: All ports except crusted port are fined using gelatin. Sherry should be treated in a similar way to wine.

COLORANTS: Cochineal (E120), produced by extracting the red body material from pregnant scale insects of the species Dactilopius Coccus, is used as a colorant in a small number of red wines, soft drinks and Campari.

CIDER

Choosing a cider that has been naturally fermented and fined can be a bit of a minefield. Producers often tend to add rather nasty clarifying agents such as gelatin, isinglass, chitin (crab shells) and collagen. The most popular commercial ciders such as

Woodpecker, Strongbow, Scrumpy Jack, Symonds and Taunton Cider all use animal-derived clarifying agents, and although they stress that these are removed during the final stages of production, The Vegetarian Society would nonetheless class them as unsuitable for vegetarians.

Vegetarian ciders are usually naturally fermented in large oak barrels and allowed to settle over a period of months (the longer, the better, as this not only makes the cider clearer, but also stronger!). Bentonite clay when mined and specially prepared for clarification purposes can also be used, or alternatively cellulose filter sheets.

Apart from fining agents, other additives are used in the production of keg cider, chiefly for sterilization. All those listed below are suitable for vegans & vegetarians:

CALCIUM SULPHITE (CALCIUM SALT OF SULPHUROUS ACID) (E226): Used as a cask sterilizer and anti-bacterial agent.

CITRIC ACID (E330): Occurs naturally in many fruits, especially citrus juices. Used to aid the effect of the anti-oxidant used.

L-ASCORBIC ACID (E300): Occurs naturally in many fruits and vegetables. Used in keg draught cider and bottled cider.

PECTOLASE: A naturally occurring enzyme used to destroy residual Pectin (a fruit starch) in keg and bottled cider.

SODIUM DIOXIDE (E220): Used as a preservative in the cask or bottle.

SODIUM HYDROGEN SULPHITE (SODIUM SALT OF SULPHUROUS ACID) (E222): Also used as a preservative and as a cask sterilizer.

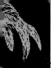

SODIUM METABISULPHITE (COMMERCIALLY MANU-FACTURED SODIUM SALT OF SULPHUROUS ACID) (E223): Used to sterilize apple skins when cultured yeast is used.

SORBIC ACID (E200): Occurs naturally in some fruits. Used as a pH adjuster.

INGREDIENTS THAT ARE USUALLY ANIMAL DERIVED

A

Acetaldehyde – Ethanol

Acetic Acid – Butyl Acetate; Butyl Ester

Acetic Anhydride – Acetyl Oxide; Acetic Oxide

Acetoin – Acetyl Methyl Carbinol

Acetyl Oxide – Acetic Anhydride; Acetic Oxide

Acetylated Sucrose Distearte

Acetylmethylcarbinol

Alanine

Alcloxa – Aluminum Chlorohydroxy Allantoinate

Aldol

Allantoin

Allantoin Acetyl Methionine

Allantoin Ascorbate

Allantoin Biotin

Allantoin Calcium Pantothenate

Allantoin Galacturonic Acid

Allantoin Glycyrrhetinic Acid

Allantoin Polygalacturonic Acid

Allantoinate

Aluminum Acetate – Burow's Solution

Aluminum Chorhydroxy Allantoinate

Aluminum Distearate

Aluminum Isostearates/Laurates/ Stearates

Aluminum Isostearates/Myristates

Aluminum Isostearates/Palmitates

Aluminum Lactate

Aluminum Myristates/Palmitates

Aluminum Salts: Aluminum Acetate/Lanolate/ Stearate/Tri-stearate

Aluminum Stearates

Aluminum Tripalmitate/Triisostearate

Aluminum Tristearate

Aminosuccinate Acid – Aspartic Acid; DL & L Forms

Ammonium C12-15 Pareth Sulfate – Pareth-25-3 Sulfate

Ammonium Isostearate

Ammonium Myristyl Sulfate

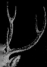

Ammonium Oleate

Ammonium Stearate –
Stearic Acid;
Ammonium Salt

Amphoteric

Amphoteric-2

Ascorbyl Stearate

Asparagine

Aspartic Acid –
DL & L Forms;
Aminosuccinate Acid

B

Basic Violet 10

Beheneth-5, -10, -20, -30

Behenic Acid – Docosanoic
Acid; Docosanol

Beta Carotene – Provitamin A

Betaine

Biotin – Vitamin H;
Vitamin B Factor

Brilliantines

Burow's Solution –
Aluminum Acetate

Butyl Acetate – Acetic Acid;
Butyl Ester

Butyl Glycolate

Butyl Oleate

Butyl Palmitate

Butyl Phrhaly Butyl Glycolate

Butylrolactone – Butanolide

C

C18-36 Acid

C29-70 Acid – C29-70
Carboxylic Acids

C18-36 Acid Glycol Ester

C18-36 Acid Triglyceride

C9-11 Alcohols

C12-16 Alcohols

C14-15 Alcohols

C12-15 Alcohols Benzoate

C12-15 Alcohols Lactate

C21 Dicarboxylic Acid

C15-18 Glycol

C18-20 Glycol Palmitate

C8-9, C9-11; C9-13; C9-14;
C10-11; C10-13; C11-12;
C11-13; C12-14;

C13-14, C13-16; and C20-40
IsoParaffins

C11-15 Pareth-12 Stearate

C11-15 Pareth-40

C12-13 Pareth 3-7

C14-15 Pareth-7, -11, -13

C10-18 Triglycerides

Calcium Stearate

Calcium Stearoyl Lactylate

Capric – Caprylic; Stearic
Triglyceride

Caproamphoacetate

Caproamphodiacetate

Capryl Betaine
Caprylamine Oxide
Caprylic; Capric; Stearic
    Triglyceride
Caprylic Acid
Caprylamphoacetate
Capryloamphodiacetate
Carbamide – Urea
Carnpxylic Acid – Deceth 7
Cetearalkonium Bromide
Ceteareth-3 – Cetyl/Stearyl
    Ether
Ceteareth-4, -6, -8, -10, -12, -15,
    -17, -20, -27, -30
Ceteareth-5
Cetaryl Alcohol
Ceteth-1
Cetyl
Cetyl Alcohol
Cetyl Ammonium
Cetyl Arachidate
Cetyl Betaine
Cetyl Esters
Cetyl Lactate
Cetyl Myristate
Cetyl Octanoate
Cetyl Palmitate
Cetyl Phosphate
Cetyl Ricinoleate
Cetyl Stearate
Cetyl Stearyl Glycol

Cetylarachidol
Cetylpyridinium Chloride
Cetyltrimethylammonium
    Bromide Chitin
Cloflucarbon

D

Deceth-7-Carboxylic Acid
Decyl Betaine
Diacetyl
Diazo
Diazolidinyl Urea –
    Germall II™
Dicetyl Adipate
Dicetyl Thiodipropionate
Diethyl Asparate
Diethyl Palmitoyl Apartate
Diethyl Sebacate
Diethylaminoethyl Stearamide
Diethylaminoethyl Stearate
Diglyceryl Stearate Malate
Dihydroxyethyl Soyamine
    Dioleate
Dihydroxyethyl Stearamine
    Oxide
Dihydroxyethyl Stearyl
    Glycinate
Dimethyl Behenamine
Dimethyl Lauramine Oleate
Dimethyl Myristamine
Dimethyl Palmitamine

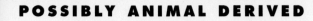

Dimethyl Stearamine

Dimethylaminopropyl
Oleamide

Dimethylaminopropyl
Stearamide

Dimethylol Urea

Dimyristyl Thiodipropionate

Dioleth-8-Phosphate

Direct Black 51

Direct Red 23 – Fast Scarlet
4BSA.

Direct Red 80

Direct Violet 48

Direct Yellow 12 –
Chrysophenine G

Disodium Cetaeryl
Sulfosuccinate

Disodium Isostearamino
Mea-Sulfosuccinate

Disodium
Monooleamidosulfosuccinate

Disodium Monoricinoleamido
MEA-Sulfosuccinate

Disodium Oleamido MIPA-
Sulfosuccinate

Disodium Oleamido PEG-2
Sulfosuccinate

Disodium Oleyl Sulfosuccinate

Disodium Stearmido
MEA-Sulfosuccinate

Disodium Stearminodipionate

Disodium Stearyl
Sulfosuccinate

Distearyl Thiodipropionate

DI-TEA-Palmitoyl Asparate

Dodecanedionic Acid; Cetearyl
Alcohol; Glycol Copolymer

Dodecyltetradecanol

E

E153

E431

E472(b)

E478

E570

E161(g)

E432

E472(c)

E479(b)

E572

E252

E433

E472(d)

E481

E585

E270

E434

E472(e)

E482

E631

E322

E435

E472(f)
E483
E635
E325
E436
E473
E491
E640
E326
E470(a)
E474
E492
E920
E327
E470(b)
E475
E493
E422
E471
E476
E494
E430
E472(a)
E477
E4951
Enfleurage
Enzyme
Ethyl Aspartate
Ethyl Oleate
Ethyl Palmitate
Ethyl Serinate

Ethyl Stearate
Ethyl Urocanate
Ethylene Dioleamide
Ethylene Distearamide
Ethylene Urea
Ethylhexyl Palmitate

F

Fatty Alcohols – Cetyl;
    Stearyl; Lauryl; Myristyl
Folic Acid
Fructose

G

Gel (not Silica gel)
Glucose Glutamate
Glyceryl Caprate
Glyceryl Caprylate
Glyceryl Caprylate/Caprate
Glyceryl Dioleate
Glyceryl Distearate
Glyceryl Hydrostearate
Glyceryl Hydroxystearate
Glyceryl Isostearate
Glyceryl Monostearate
Glyceryl Myristate
Glyceryl Oleate
Glyceryl Palmitate Lactate
Glyceryl Stearate SE
Glyceryl Trimyristate
Glycol Stearate SE

Glycyrrhetinyl Stearate
Guanidine Carbonate
Guanosine

H

Hexanediol Distearate
Histidine
Hydrogenated
    Fatty Oils
Hydroxylated Lecithin
Hydroxyoctacosanyl
    Hydroxyastearate
Hydroxystearmide MEA
Hydroxystearic Acid

I

Imidazlidinyl Urea,
Indole
Isobutyl Myristate
Isobutyl Palmitate
Isobutyl Stearate
Isoceteth-10, -20, -30
Isocetyl Alcohol
Isocetyl Isodecanoate
Isocetyl Palmitate
Isocetyl Stearate
Isocetyl Stearoyl
    Stearate
Isoceteth-10 Stearate
Isodecyl Hydroxystearate
Isodecyl Myristate

Isodecyl Oleate
Isodecyl Palmitate
Isohyxyl Palmitate
Isopropyl Acetate
Isopropyl Isostearate
Isopropyl Myristate
Isopropyl Palmitate
Isopropyl Stearate
Isostearamidopropalkonium
    Chloride
Isostearamidopropyl Betaine
Isostearamidopropyl
    Dimethylamine Glycolate
Isostearamidopropyl
    Dimethylamine Lactate
Isostearamidopropyl
    Ethyldimonium Ethosulfate
Isostearamidopropyl
    Morpholine Lactate
Isostearamidoporopylamine
    Oxide
Isosteareth-2 through -20
Isostearic Acid
Isostearoamphoglycinate
Isostearoamphopropionate
Isostearyl Alcohol
Isostearyl Benzylimidonium
    Chloride
Isostearyl Diglyceryl Succinate
Isostearyl Erucate
Isostearyl Ethylimidonium

Ethosulfate
Isostearyl Hydroxyethyl
Imidazoline
Isostearyl. Imidazoline
Isostearyl Isostearate
Isostearyl Lactate
Isostearyl Neopentanoate
Isostearyl Palmitate
Isostearyl Stearoyl Stearate

L

Lactic Acid
Lauroyl Sarcosine
Lauryl Isostearate
Lauryl Palmitate
Lauryl Stearate
Lauryl Suntaine
Lithium Stearate

M

Magnesium Myristate
Magnesium Oleate
Magnesium Stearate
Methyl Gluceth-10 or -20
Methyl Glucet-20
Sesquistereate – Glucamate
Methyl Glucose Sesquioleate
Methyl Glucose Sesquistearate
Methyl Hydroxystearate
Methyl Lactate
Methyl Myristate

Methyl Oleate
Methyl Palmitate
Mixed Isopropanolamines
Myristate
Morpholine Stearate
Myreth-3
Myreth-3 Caprate – Myristic
Ethoxy Caprate
Myreth-3 Laurate
Myreth-3 Myristate
Myreth-4
Myristamide DEA – Myristic
Diethanolamide
Myristamide MIPA
Myristamidopropyl Betaine
Myristamidopropyl
Diethylamine
Myristamidopropylamine
Oxide
Myristamine Oxide
Myristaminopropionic Acid
Myristate
Myristic Acid
Myristimide MEA
Myristoamphoacetate
Myristoyl Sarcosine
Myristyl Alcohol
Myristyl Betaine
Myristyl Hydroxyethyl
Imidazoline
Myristyl Isostearate

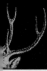
Myristyl Lactate
Myristyl Myristate
Myristyl Neopentanoate –
    Ceraphyl
Myristyl Propionate
Myristyl Stearate
Myristyleicosanol
Myristyleicosyl Stearate
Myristyloctadecanol

N

Nonyl Acetate

O

Octododecanol-2 – Octyl
    Dodecanol
Octododeceth-20, -25
Octododecyl Myristate
Octoxyglyceryl Behenate
Octyl Acetoxystearate
Octyl Hydroxystearate
Octyl Palmitate
Octyl Stearate
Octyldodecyl Stearate
Octyldodecyl Stearoyl Stearate
Oleamide – Oleylamide
Oleamide DEA – Oleic
    Diethanolamide
Oleamide MIPA
Oleamine Oxide
Oleic Acid

Oleoyl Sarcosine
Oleth-3 Phosphate
Oleth 20
Oleth-20 Phosphate
Oleyl Betaine
Oleyl Myristate
Oleyl Oleate
Oleyl Stearate
Orotic Acid –
    Pyrimidecarboxylic Acid

P

Palmamamidopropyl Betaine
Palmitamide DEA, MEA
Palmitamidopropyl Betaine
Palmitamindopropyl
    Diethylamine
Palmitamine
Palmitamine Oxide – Palmityl
    Dimethylamine Oxide
Palmitate
Palmitic Acid
Panthenyl Ethyl Etheracetate
Pareth-25-12
PEG-9 Caprylate
PEG-8 Caprylate / Caprate
PEG-6 Caprylic / Capric
    Glycerides
PEG-6 to -150 Dioleate
PEG-3 Dipalmitate
PEG-2 through -175 Distearate

PEG-5 through -120 Glyceryl
Stearate
PEG-25 Glyceryl Trioleate
PEG-6 or -12 Isostearate
PEG-20 Methyl Glucose
Sesquistearate
PEG-4 Octanoate
PEG-2 through -9 Oleamide
PEG-2 through -30 Oleamide
PEG-12, -20, or -30 Oleate
PEG-3 through -150 Oleate
PEG-6 through -20 Palmitate
PEG-25 through -125 Propylene
Glycol Stearate
PEG-8 Sesquioleate
PEG-5 or -20 Sorbitan
Isostearate
PEG-3 or -6 Sorbitan Oleate
PEG-80 Sorbitan Palmitate
PEG-40 Sorbitan Peroleate
PEG-3 or -40 Sorbitan Stearate
PEG-30, -40, or -60 Sorbitan
Tetraoleate
PEG-60 Sorbitan Tetrastearate
PEG-2 through -150 Stearate
PEG-66 or -200
Trihydroxystearin
Pentaerythrityl Tetraoctanoate
Pentaerythrityl Tetrastearate
and Calcium Stearate
Phospholipids – Phosphatides

Polyglycerol
Polyglycerol-4 Cocoate
Polyglycerol-10 Decalinoleate
Polyglycerol-2 Diisostearate
Polyglycerol-6 Dioleate
Polyglycerol-6 Distearate
Polyglycerol-3 Hydroxylauryl
Ether
Polyglycerol-4 Isostearate
Polyglycerol-3, -4 or -8 Oleate
Polyglycerol-2 or -4 Oleyl Ether
Polyglycerol-2 PEG-4 Stearate
Polyglycerol-2
Sesquiisostearate
Polyglycerol-2 Sesquioleate
Polyglycerol-3, -4 or -8 Stearate
Polyglycerol-10 Tetraoleate
Polyglycerol-2 Tetrastearate
Polysorbate 60/Polysorbate 80
Potassium Apartate
Potassium Coco-Hydrolyzed
Protein
Potassium DNA
Potassium Oleate – Oleic Acid
Potassium Salt
Potassium Myristate
Potassium Palmitate
Potassium Stearate – Stearic
Acid Potassium Salt
PPG-3-Myreth-11
PPG-4-Ceteareth-12

PPG-4-Ceteth-1, -5 or -10
PPG-4 Myristyl Ether
PPG-5-Ceteth-10 Phosphate
PPG-6-C12-18 Pareth
PPG-8-Ceteth, -5, -10, or -20
PPG-9-Steareth-3
PPG-10-Ceteareth-20
PPG-10 Cetyl Ether leyl Ether
PPG-11 or -15 Stearyl Ether
PPG-26 Oleate –
    Polyoxypropylene 2000
    Monooleate; Carbowax
PPG-28 Cetyl Ether
PPG-30 Cetyl Ether
PPG-30,-50, Oleyl, Ether
PPG-36 Oleate –
    Polyoxypropylene (36)
    Monooleate
PPG-Isocetyl Ether PPG-3-
    Isosteareth-9
Proline
Propylene Glycol Myristate
Protein Fatty Acid
    Condensates
Proteins
Pyridium Compounds
Pyroligneous Acid

R

Retinyl Palmitate
Ribonucleic Acid – RNA

S

Sarcosines
S-Carboxy Methyl Cysteine
Sebactic Acid – Decanedioic
    Acid
Serine
Skatole
Sodium Aluminum
    Chlorohydroxy Lactate
Sodium C12-15 Pareth-7
    Carboxylate
Sodium C12-15 Pareth-Sulfate
Sodium Cetearyl Sulfate
Sodium Cetyl Sulfate
Sodium Cocyl Sarcosinate
Sodium DNA
Sodium Glyceryl Oleate
    Phosphate
Sodium Isosteareth-6
    Carboxylate
Sodium Isosteroyl Lacrylate
Sodium Myreth Sulfate
Sodium Myristate
Sodium Myristoyl Isethionate
Sodium Myristoyl Sarcosinate
Sodium Myristyl Sulfate
Sodium Oleth-7 or -8
    Phosphate
Sodium Palmitate
Sodium Pareth-15-7 or 25-7

Carboxylate
Sodium Pareth-23 or -25 Sulfate
Sodium PCA
Sodium PCA Methysilanol
Sodium Ribonucleic Acid –
  SRNA
Sodium Sarcosinate
Sodium Soap
Sodium Stearate
Sodium Steroyl Lactylate
Sodium Urocanate
Sorbeth-6 Hexastearate
Sorbitan Diisoseate
Sorbitan Dioleate
Sorbitan Fatty Acid Esters
Sorbitan Isostearate
Sorbitan Oleate – Sorbitan
  Monooleate
Sorbitan Palmitate –
  Span 40™
Sorbitan Sesquioleate
Sorbitan Sequistearate
Sorbitan Triisostearate
Sorbitan Tristearate
Spermaceti – Cetyl Palmitate
Stearalkonium Bentonite
Stearalkonium Chloride
Stearalkonium Hectorite
Stearamide
Stearamide DEA – Stearic Acid
  Diethanolamide

Stearamide DIBA Stearate
Stearamide MIPA
Stearamide MIPA Stearate
Stearamide Oxide
Stearmidopropalkonium
  Chloride
Stearamidopropyl
  Dimethylamine
Stearamine
Stearamine Oxide
Stearates
Steareth-2
Steareth-4 through -100
Stearic Acid
Stearic Hydrazide
Stearmidoethyl Diethylamine
Stearoamphoacetate
Stearoamphocarboxyglycinate
Stearoamphodiacetate
Stearoamphohydroxypropysulf
  onate
Stearoamphopropionate
Stearone
Stearoxy Dimethicone
Stearoxytrimethylsilane
Stearoyl Lactylic Acid
Stearoyl Sarcosine
Steartrimonium Chloride
Steartrimonium Hydrolyzed
  Animal Protein
Stearyl Acetate

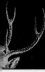

Stearyl Betaine
Stearyl Caprylate
Stearyl Citrate
Stearyl Erucamide
Stearyl Erucate
Stearyl Ghycyrrhetinate
Stearyl Heptanoate
Stearyl Hydroxyethyl
　Imidazoline
Stearyl Lactate
Stearyl Octanoate
Stearyl Stearate
Stearyl Stearoyl Stearate
Stearyldimethyl Amine
Stearylvinyl Ether/Maleic
　Anhydride Copolymer
Steroids
Stenol
Sterol
Sucrose Distearate
Sucrose Laurate
Sucrose Stearate
Synthetic Spermaceti

T

TEA-Lauroyl Sarcosinate
TEA-Myristate
TEA-Oleate – Triethanolamine
　Oleate
TEA-Palm-Kernel Sarcosinate
TEA-Stearate

Terpinyl Acetate
Tetramethyl
　Decynediol
TIPA-Stearate
Tridecyl Stearate
Trihydroxy Stearin
Triisostearin
Trimethylopropane
　Triisostearate
Trimyristin-Glyceryl
　Trimyristate
Trioleth-8 Phosphate
Trioleyl Phosphate
Tristearin
Tristearyl Citrate
Tryptophan
Tyrosine

U

Undecylpentadecanol
Urea – Carbamide
Urease

V

Valine

W

Waxes

Z

Zinc Stearate – Zinc Soa

CHAPTER 1: **THINGS TO KNOW**

WHERE DID THE TERM "VEGETARIAN" COME FROM?
From the Internet:
www.vegsource.com/articles/veg_definition.htm
www.vegan.org/FAQs/index.html

COMMON MYTHS
From The Internet: www.vegan.org/FAQs/index.html
Proctor & Gamble
Center for Science in the Public Interest (CSPI)

OLESTRA®
Proctor & Gamble
Center for Science in the Public Interest (CSPI)

ON KOSHER...
Kosher Information Web Site:
jewishveg.com/schwartz/dietlaws.html

WAXED PRODUCE
The Bread & Circus Whole Food Bible, Christopher Kilham;
Addison Wesley, 1991.
The Complete Book of Juicing, Michael Murray, ND; Prima
Publishing, 1992.

CHAPTER 2: **VEGAN NUTRIENTS**

*The Vegan Diet as Chronic Disease Prevention: Evidence Supporting
the New Four Food Groups*, Kerrie K. Saunders, Ph.D.
*A Brief Introduction To Basic Nutrition. Adapted from Basic
Nutrition*, The Vegetarian Society UK.
Soy Not Oi, Hippycore; AK Press.
The Nutrition Bible, Jean Anderson, MS & Barbara Deskins, PhD, RD.

Minimax, Dr. David Phillips.
Vegan Delights, Eva Batt; Thorsons.
Bantam Medical Dictionary; Bantam.
Recommended Dietary Allowances, 10th ed., The Food and Nutrition Board, National Research Council; National Academy Press, 1989.
Simply Vegan: Quick Vegetarian Meals, Debra Wasserman and Reed Mangels, PhD, RD; The Vegetarian Resource Group.
Basic Nutrition Information Sheet, The Vegetarian Society UK.

CHAPTER 3: DEFINITIVE LISTINGS

ANIMAL INGREDIENTS AND THEIR ALTERNATIVES.
Animal Factories, Jim Mason; Crown Publishers.
Center for Science in the Public Interest (CSPI).
Product Labels.
Slaughter of the Innocent, Hans Ruesch.
List Of Animal Products and Their Alternatives, Jon Cardillo.
Animal Liberation, Peter Singer; Avon.
A Consumer's Dictionary of Cosmetic Ingredients, Ruth Winter; Crown.
From The Internet:
www.peta.org/mall/cc/ingred1.html
www.peta.org/mall/cc/ingred.html
Assorted information from VegSocUK.

CHAPTER 4: ANIMAL INGREDIENTS

Personal Care with Principle, National Anti-Vivisection Society.
E.G. Smith Collective Research.
Center for Science in the Public Interest (CSPI).

CHAPTER 5: ALCOHOL

"Ask the Bay Vegan," *The Bay Vegan*, No. 4, Summer 1996.

BITTERS, ETC
"Beer," VegSocUK Info Sheet

LOW ALCOHOL
"Beer," VegSocUK Info Sheet.
"Cruelty-Free Beers," *Animal-Times*, Jan/Feb 1995; PETA.

LAGERS
"Beer," VegSocUK Info Sheet.

US DOMESTIC
Manufacturer Contacts.
Product Labels.
Common Sense.
"Cruelty-Free Beers," *Animal-Times*, Jan/Feb 1995; PETA.
"This list is not intended to be exhaustive, and inclusion on the list is not an endorsement of the producer or manufacturer. PETA makes no claim regarding these companies' environmental, business, or advertising practices." (Uhh, nor does E.G. Smith Press)
* Coors products intentionally deleted from list.

VEGAN WINES
"Alcohol," VegSocUK Info Sheet.

OUTSIDE THE US
"Alcohol," VegSocUK Info Sheet.

CIDER
"Cider," VegSocUK Info Sheet.

CHAPTER 6: POSSIBLY ANIMAL DERIVED

E.G. Smith Collective Research
Center for Science in the Public Interest (CSPI)

SOURCES, RESOURCES & CONTACTS

"Personal Care with Principle," National Anti-Vivisection Society, Spring, 1992.

ADDRESSES AND PHONE NUMBERS

UNITED STATES:

American Vegan Society
56 Dinshah Lane, P.O. Box 369, Malaga NJ 08328
(856) 694-2887
www.americanvegan.org

Vegan Action
PO Box 4288
Richmond, VA 23220
(804) 502-8736
www.vegan.org/FAQs/index.html

North American Vegetarian Society (NAVS)
PO Box 72 Dolgeville, NY 13329
(518) 568-7970
E-mail: mailto:navs@telenet.net
www.navs-online.org/

The Vegetarian Resource Group (VRG)
P.O. Box 1463, Dept. IN
Baltimore, MD 21203
(410) 366-VEGE
Email: mailto:vrg@vrg.org
www.vrg.org/nutshell/about.htm

People for the Ethical Treatment of Animals (PETA)
501 Front Street
Norfolk, VA 23510
(757) 622-PETA • www.peta.org

Vegetarian Resource Network
Post Office Box 321
Knoxville, TN 37901-0321
(800) USA-VEGE
www.veganet.com

VegNews
PO Box 320130
San Francisco, CA 94132
(415) 665.NEWS
www.vegnews.com

EUROPEAN:

European Vegetarian Union (EVU)
Vondelstraat 9A2, NL-1054 GB
Amsterdam, The Netherlands
tel/fax: 0031-206169146 • email: evueuro@worldaccess.nl

Information and Contacts in Europe:

Denmark:
Henrik Hedegard, Olivenvej 57, DK-6000 Kolding

Belgium:
Vegetariersbond vzw, Koewacht 16A, B-9190 Stekene

Finland:
Elavan Ravinnon Yhdistys Ry., Kasarminkatu 19A, SF-00130 Helsinki

France:
Jean Montagard, Chemin Combe Nicette, F-06330 Roquefort-les-Pins
Gertrud Krueger, Rue Brandmatt 22, F-68380 Metzeral

Italy:
Associazione Vegetariana Italiana, Via Bazzini 4, I-20131 Milano

Lithuania:
Eduardas Mickevicius, Antakalnio 67-17, LIT-2040 Vilnius

Netherlands:
Nederlandse Vegetariersbond, Larenseweg 26, NL-1221 CM Hilversum
Netherlands Nederlandse Vereiniging voor Veganisme, Postbus 1087, NL-6801 BB, Arnheim

Ireland:
Vegetarian Society of Ulster, 66 Ravenshill Gardens, Ballynafeigh, Belfast

Norway:
Norges Vegetariske Landsvorbun, Munkedamsveien 3B, N-0161 Oslo1

Austria:
Oestereichische Vegetarier-Union, E. Laupert, Brucknerstrasse 59/18, A 8010 Graz

Poland:
Krystyna Chomicz-Jung, Gdanska 2m.97, PL-01-633 Warszaw

Romania:
Dr. Mircea Matusan, Str. Costei no 12, RO-3400 Cluj-Napoca

Russia:
Tatyana Pavlova, Volsky bulvar d39 k3 kv23, RUS-109462 Moscow

Sweden:
Vegetariska Foreningen, Box 4256, S-10266 Stockholm
Ulla Troeng, Klovervagen 6, S-61700 Mariefred

Switzerland:
"regeneration" Edwin Heller, Schwarzenbachweg 16, CH 8049 Zurich

Schweizer Verein f. Vegetarismus, Renato Pichler, Postfach, CH-9466, Sennwald

Slovakia:
Vegetarianska spolocnost, Prazka 9, SK-81104 Bratislava

Spain:
Spanish Vegan Society, Apartado Postal 38127, E-28080 Madrid

CRUELTY-FREE PRODUCTS/INFORMATION

PETA Mall: www.petamall.com/index.html
Pangea Vegan Products ("For a Cruelty-Free Lifestyle"):
    www.veganstore.com
Animal Rights Stuff:www.animalrightsstuff.com
Seventh Generation (cleaning products)
Shop At Ethics: www.shopatethics.biz
The Vegetarian Site: www.thevegetariansite
Vegan Essentials: www.veganessentials.com
Vegan Mercantile: www.veganmercantile.com
Vegan Street: www.veganstreet.com
The Vegan Society (prices listed in pounds):
    www.vegansociety.com/catalog/default.php
Vegan Wares (vegan shoes from Autralia): www.veganwares.com
Moo Shoes (vegan shoes and accessories): www.mooshoes.com
NoMeat.com ("the vegetarian meat substitute online grocer"):
    www.nomeat.com
Vegan Companion Animal Food: www.vegancats.com
Long list of vegan companies:
    www.hedweb.com/campaig/vegcomp.htm
Imagine Foods: www.imaginefoods.com/pages/info/vegan.html

Vegan Shoes in the UK: www.veganline.com
Nice long list of UK shops & sites:
    www.veganvillage.co.uk/shops.htm
Snooty Jewelry (vegan jewelry):
    www.snootyjewelry.com/index.htm
Different Daisy (vegan products): www.differentdaisy.com
Ginny's Vegan Ready-Made Food:
    ginnysveganfoods.com/index.html
Lightlife Foods: www.lightlife.com/index.html
Roads End Organics (vegan cheese): www.chreese.com

MAIL ORDER BOOK OUTLETS

AK Press (U.S.)
674-A 23rd Street, Oakland, CA 94612
(510) 208-1700 • fax: (510) 208-1701
email: akpress@akpress.org • www.akpress.org

AK Press (Eurpoe)
P.O. Box 12766, Edinburgh, Scotland, EH8 9YE
(0131) 555-5165 • fax: (0131) 555-5215
email: ak@akedin.demon.co.uk • www.akuk.com

Vegetarian Resource Group
P.O. Box 1463 Dept. IN, Baltimore, MD 21203
(410)366-VEGE
www.vrg.org/nutshell/about.htm

RECOMMENDED LITERATURE

COOKBOOKS
The Vegan Cookbook, Alan Wakeman and Gordon Baskerville;
London, Faber and Faber, 1986. This has basic as well as complex
stuff.

Friendly Foods, Brother Ron Pickarski; Berkeley, Ten Speed, 1991. Vegan.

Laurel's Kitchen: A Handbook for Vegetarian Cookery and Nutrition, Laurel Robertson, Carol Flinders, and Bronwen Godfrey; Nilgiri Press.

Moosewood (all selections), The Moosewood Collective; Simon and Schuster.

The Complete Vegetarian Cuisine, Rose Elliot; Pantheon Books. Many dishes are vegan.

Fast Vegetarian Feasts, Martha Rose Shulman; Doubleday.

Tassajara Cooking, Richard Bakerroshi; Shambhala. Cooking made simple!

The Vegetarian Epicure I and II, Anna Thomas; Knopf.

American Whole Foods Cookbook.

How to Overthrow Any Government Without Violence Cookbook, James P. Martin. Vegan.

The Joy of Cooking Naturally, Peggy Dameron. Vegan, includes honey.

Country Life Vegetarian Cookbook, Diana J. Fleming, ed.

Of These Ye May Eat Freely, special nightshade-free section.

Cooking from an Italian Garden, Paola Scaravelli; Holt, Rinehart, and Winston.

The Cranks Cookbook, Cranks (London restaurant).

The Findhorn Cookbook, Barbara Friedlander; feeds 1 to 100.

The Apartment Vegetarian Cookbook, Lindsay Miller; Peace Press.

Back to Eden, Jethro Kloss; Back to Eden Books. Definitive herb book with recipes.

Bean Banquets: From Boston to Bombay, Patricia R. Gregory; Woodbridge Press.

Eat More, Weigh Less, Dean Ornish, M.D.; Harper Collins.

NON-FICTION

Diet for a New America, John Robbins; Stillpoint.

Animal Liberation, Peter Singer; Avon.

The MacDougal Plan and The MacDougal Program.

A Vegetarian Sourcebook, Keith Akers; Putnam.

Vegan Nutrition: Pure and Simple, Michael Klaper, M.D.; Gentle World, Inc.

Pregnancy, Children, and the Vegan Diet, Michael Klaper, M.D.; Gentle World, Inc.

Simply Vegan, Debra Wasserman; Vegetarian Resource Group.

The Vegan Diet as Chronic Disease Prevention, Kerrie K. Saunders, Lantern Books.

TRAVEL & RESTAURANT RESOURCES

The Vegan Guide to New York City, Max Friedman, 2231 McKinley St., Berkeley, CA 94703. A detailed directory of reviews to more than 100 restaurants in Manhattan and Brooklyn serving delicious meals without any animal products. To order: $4.78 (USA) or $8.00 (world).

Vegetarian Journal's Guide to Natural Foods Restaurants in the U.S. and Canada, The Vegetarian Resource Group. Lists restaurants, vacation spots, camps, vegetarian organizations.

The Vegan Holiday and Restaurant Guide, NAVS, PO Box 72, Dolgeville, NY 13329. Focused on England, Scotland and Wales, $18 (USA) or $21 (world).

Vegetarian Gourmet, Chitra Publications, 2 Public Avenue, Montrose, PA

The Vegan, The Vegan Society, 7 Battle Road, St Leonards-on-Sea, East Sussex TN37, 7AA, UK

Ahimsa, American Vegan Society, 56 Dinshah Lane, PO Box 369, Malaga, NJ 08328, (856) 694-2887

Vegetarian Journal, Vegetarian Resource Group, PO. Box 1463, Dept. IN, Baltimore, MD 21203, (410) 366-8343

Vegetarian Living, HHL Publishing Group Ltd, Greater London House, Hampstead Rd, London NW1 7QQ, UK

BBC Vegetarian Good Food Guide, P.O. Box 425, Woking GU21 1GP, UK

ANIMAL RIGHTS ORGANIZATIONS

Humane Society of the US
2100 " L" Street NW. Washington, DC 20037
Posters against animal research available.

FARM (Farm Animal Reform Movement)
PO. Box 70123, Washington, DC 20088
(301) 530-1737
Publishes quarterly newsletter and informational handouts.

PETA (People for the Ethical Treatment of Animals)
P.O. Box 42516, Washington, DC 20015
Publishes Cruelty-free Shopping Guide and other informational literature.

National Anti-Vivisection Society
53 W. Jackson Blvd., Suite 1550, Chicago, IL 60604
(312) 427-6065
Free cruelty-free products listing.

SOURCES OF INFORMATION ON THE INTERNET

General veg sites listing:
   www.mit.edu/activities/vsg/links.shtml
List of animal ingredients:
   members.aol.com/docvegan/_animalingredients.html
General vegan site:
   www.Vegan.com

2:15, HELLO

A Map of Heaven, HENRY NORMAL

Addicted To War, JOEL ANDREAS

Anarchism, Marxism, and the Future of the Left, MURRAY BOOKCHIN

Anarchism: Arguments For & Against (2nd), ALBERT MELTZER

Anarcho-Syndicalism, RUDOLF ROCKER

Anarchy in the UK: The Angry Brigade, TOM VAGUE

Animal Ingredients A to Z (3rd edition), E.G. SMITH COLLECTIVE

Assault on Culture, STEWART HOME

At War With Asia, NOAM CHOMSKY

Bad, JAMES CARR

Beat the Heat: How to Handle Encounters with Law Enforcement,
    KATYA KOMISARUK

Beggars of Life, JIM TULLY

Beneath the Paving Stones, DARK STAR COLLECTIVE

A Cavalier History Of Surrealism, A, RAOUL VANEIGEM

Complete Cinematic Works of Guy Debord, KEN KNABB

Controlled Flight Into Terrain, JOHN YATES

Crass Art and Other Pre Post-Modernist Manifestos, GEE VOUCHER

Critical Mass: Bicycling's Defiant Celebration,
    ED. By CHRIS CARLSSON

Diamond Signature, PENNY RIMBAUD

Direct Action: Memoirs of an Urban Guerilla, ANN HANSEN

Dream Ticket, HENRY NORMAL

Ecofascism, JANET BIEHL & PETER STAUDENMAIER

End Time 2nd edition, G.A. MATIASZ

Excite the Mind, VARIOUS

Facing the Enemy: A History of Anarchist Organization
from Proudhon to May '68, ALEXANDRE SKIRDA

Fifteenth of February, HENRY NORMAL

Four Letter World, DAN O'MAHONY

Free Women of Spain, MARTHA ACKELSBERG

Friends Of Durruti Group, 1937—1939, The,
AGUSTAN GUILLAMON

Great British Mistake, The, TOM VAGUE

Housing Benefit Hill & Other Places, CJ STONE

I Couldn't Paint Golden Angels, ALBERT MELTZER

Idol Killing, An, MARK J. WHITE

Immediatism, HAKIM BEY

Jumping the Line, WILLIAM HERRICK

Language and Politics, NOAM CHOMSKY

Legacy to Liberation, ED. FRED HO

Pie any Means Necessary, ED. AGENT APPLE

Little Book of Vegan Poems, BENJAMIN ZEPHANIAH

Memoirs of Vidocq: Master of Crime,
FRANCOIS EUGENE VIDOCQ

Moving Forward: Program for a Participatory Economy,
MICHAEL ALBERT

Neoism, Plagiarism & Praxis, STEWART HOME

Neoist Manifestos / The Art Strike Papers, STEWART HOME

Nestor Mahkno–Anarchy's Cossack, ALEXANDRE SKIRDA

New World in Our Hearts: 8 Years of Writings from
the Love & Rage Revolutionary Anarchist Federation,
ED. ROY SAN FILIPPO

No Gods No Masters:An Anthology of Anarchism, Book One,
    ED. DANIEL GUERIN
No Gods No Masters: An Anthology of Anarchism, Book Two,
    ED. DANIEL GUERIN
No Pity, STEWART HOME
Obsolete Communism: The Left-Wing Alternative,
    DANIEL & GABRIEL COHN-BENDIT
Orgasms of History: 3000 Years of Spontaneous Revolt,
    YVES FREMION & VOLNY
Out of the Night, JAN VALTIN
Philosophy Of Punk, The, CRAIG OHARA
Politics of Anti-Semitism, ED. COCKBURN And ST.CLAIR
Poll Tax Rebellion, DANNY BURNS
Pussycat Fever, KATHY ACKER
Quiet Rumours: An Anarcha-Feminist Reader,
    DARK STAR COLLECTIVE
Radical Priorities, NOAM CHOMSKY
Rage and Reason, MICHAEL TOBIAS
Reading Capital Politically, HARRY CLEAVER
Realization & Suppression of the Situationists, SIMON FORD
Rebel Moon, NORMAN NAWROCKI
Red London, STEWART HOME
On the Justice of Roosting Chickens, WARD CHURCHILL
Reinventing Anarchy, Again, ED. HOWARD J. EHRLICH
Sabate: Guerilla Extraordinary, ANTONIO TELLEZ
School's Out, BENJAMIN ZEPHANIAH
Scum Manifesto, VALERIE SOLANAS

Seizing the Airwaves, RON SAKOLSKY & STEPHEN DUNIFER

September Commando, JOHN YATES

Serpents in the Garden, ED. COCKBURN AND ST.CLAIR

Shibboleth, PENNY RIMBAUD

Siege Of Gresham, RAY MURPHY

Sister of the Road, DR. BEN REITMAN

Social Anarchism Or Lifestyle Anarchism:
    An Unbridgeable Chasm, MURRAY BOOKCHIN

Some Recent Attacks, JAMES KELMAN

Spanish Anarchists: The Heroic Years 1868–1936, The,
    MURRAY BOOKCHIN

Struggle Against The State & Other Essays, NESTOR MAKHNO

Tales From the Clit, ED. CHERIE MATRIX

Televisionaries, TOM VAGUE

Test Card F, ANONYMOUS

Third Person, HENRY NORMAL

To Remember Spain: The Anarchist and Syndicalist Revolution
    of 1936, MURRAY BOOKCHIN

Ulster's White Negroes, FIONBARRA O'DOCHARTAIGH

Unfinished Business, CLASS WAR FEDERATION

Urban Love Poetry, HENRY NORMAL

Voltarine DeCleyre Reader, VOLTAIRINE DE CLEYRE

What is Anarchism?, ALEXANDER BERKMAN

What Is Situationism? A Reader, STEWART HOME

Which Way for the Ecology Movement?, MURRAY BOOKCHIN

Workers' Councils, ANTON PANNEKOEK

You Can't Win, 2nd edition, JACK BLACK

Spoken Word/Music CD's from AK Press:

1936 The Spanish Revolution, THE EX

175 Progress Drive, MUMIA ABU JAMAL

All Things Censored Vol.1, MUMIA ABU JAMAL

American Addiction, An, NOAM CHOMSKY

Artists In A Time of War, HOWARD ZINN

Beating the Devil, ALEXANDER COCKBURN

Become the Media, JELLO BIAFRA

Behind the Barricades: Best of David Rovics, DAVID ROVICS

Better Read Than Dead, VARIOUS

Beyond The Valley of the Gift Police, JELLO BIAFRA

Case Studies in Hypocrisy, NOAM CHOMSKY

Chile: Promise of Freedom, FREEDOM ARCHIVES

Class War, NOAM CHOMSKY

Clinton Vision, NOAM CHOMSKY

Come September, ARUNDHATI ROY

Doing Time: The Politics of Imprisonment, WARD CHURCHILL

Emerging Framework of World Power, NOAM CHOMSKY

For A Free Humanity: For Anarchy,
        NOAM CHOMSKY/CHUMBAWUMBA

Free Market Fantasies, NOAM CHOMSKY

Heroes and Martyrs, HOWARD ZINN

High Priest of Harmful Matter, JELLO BIAFRA

I Blow Minds For A Living, JELLO BIAFRA

I've Got To Know, UTAH PHILIPS

If Evolution Is Outlawed, JELLO BIAFRA

In A Pig's Eye: Reflections on the Police State,
        Repression and Native America, WARD CHURCHILL

Less Rock, More Talk, VARIOUS
Life in Occupied America, WARD CHURCHILL
Machine Gun In The Clown's Hand, JELLO BIAFRA
Mob Action Against the State: Collected, VARIOUS
Monkeywrenching the New World Order, VARIOUS
Mumia Abu-Jamal/Man is the Bastard , MUMIA ABU JAMAL
New War On Terrorism: Fact And Fiction, NOAM CHOMSKY
No More Cocoons, JELLO BIAFRA
Nora's Place and Other Poems 1965—99, TOM LEONARD
Pacifism and Pathology in the American Left, WARD CHURCHILL
People's History of the United States, HOWARD ZINN
People's History Project Boxed Set, HOWARD ZINN
Prison Industrial Complex, The, ANGELA DAVIS
Prisons On Fire: Attica, George Jackson and Black Liberation,
    GEORGE JACKSON
Propaganda and Control of the Public Mind, NOAM CHOMSKY
Prospects for Democracy, NOAM CHOMSKY
Return of the Read Menace, VARIOUS
Seven Stories, JAMES KELMAN
Stories Hollywood Never Tells, HOWARD ZINN
Taking Liberties, CHRISTIAN PARRENTI
Who Bombed Judi Bari?, JUDI BARI
Read Army Faction, VARIOUS

DVDs from AK Press
Distorted Morality , NOAM CHOMSKY
Instant Mix Imperial Democracy, ARUNDHATI ROY

ORDERING INFORMATION ON FOLLOWING PAGE

AK PRESS U.S.

674-A 23rd Street,
Oakland, CA 94612-1163
USA

Phone: (510) 208-1700
E-mail: akpress@akpress.org
www.akpress.org
Please send all payments (checks, money orders, or cash at your
own risk) in U.S. dollars. Alternatively, we take VISA and MC.

AK PRESS EUROPE

PO Box 12766,
Edinburgh, EH8 9YE
Scotland

Phone: (0131) 555-5165
E-mail: ak@akedin.demon.uk
www.akuk.com
Please send all payments (cheques, money orders, or cash at your
own risk) in U.K. pounds. Alternatively, we take credit cards.

For a dollar, a pound or a few IRC's, the same addresses would be
delighted to provide you with the latest complete AK catalog, fea-
turing several thousand books, pamphlets, zines, audio products
and stylish apparel published & distributed by AK Press.
Alternatively, check out our websites for the complete catalog, latest news and updates, events, and secure ordering.